Abs
on the
Ball

Also by Colleen Craig

*Pilates on the Ball: The World's Most Popular Workout
Using the Exercise Ball*

Abs
on the
Ball

A Pilates Approach
to Building
Superb Abdominals

Colleen Craig

Healing Arts Press
Rochester, Vermont

Healing Arts Press
One Park Street
Rochester, Vermont 05767
www.InnerTraditions.com

Healing Arts Press is a division of Inner Traditions International

Note to the reader: This book is intended as an informational guide. The remedies, approaches, and techniques described herein are meant to supplement, and not to be a substitute for, professional medical care or treatment. They should not be used to treat a serious ailment without prior consultation with a qualified health care professional.

Library of Congress Cataloging-in-Publication Data
Craig, Colleen.
    Abs on the ball : A Pilates approach to building superb abdominals / Colleen Craig.
        p. cm.
    ISBN 0-89281-098-X
    1. Bodybuilding. 2. Pilates method. 3. Swiss exercise balls. I. Title.
    GV546.5.C73 2003
    646.7'5—dc21

                                                              2003003760

Printed and bound in the Canada by Transcontinental Printing

10   9   8   7   6   5   4

Text design by Cindy Sutherland
Text layout by Virginia Scott Bowman
This book was typeset in Goudy with Avant Garde as the display typeface

Contents

1

Why Another Book on Abdominal Conditioning?

We all understand why some instruction is necessary when we are learning to drive a car for the first time, or operate a computer, or speak a new language. The same applies to abdominal conditioning, even though we use our bodies every day with no "instruction manual." If we want to tone our abdominals effectively and receive the benefits of a sturdy low back and optimal posture, we have to teach our deep muscles to work properly. *Abs on the Ball* is about training the endurance capacity of the stabilizing muscles of the abdomen and back from the inside out. This book will give you the information you need, whatever your level of fitness, to build superb abdominal strength and a healthy back.

Some of the principles introduced here may be new to you. Whether you are a professional athlete, a seasoned fitness buff, or a novice launching into your first workout, it is important to start slowly and carefully with the Fundamental Exercises at the beginning of each practice chapter in order to benefit fully from *Abs on the Ball*. But before we begin it is worth asking: Why another book on abdominal conditioning? What is wrong with the techniques we learned in the past? And what is so special about working out with a ball?

The Problem with Traditional "Ab Conditioning"

Every time I visit a gym, attend a fitness class, or watch athletes train I see examples of poor technique, unbalanced bodies, and faulty movement patterns, but nowhere is there more misunderstanding than in abdominal training. People perform endless sit-ups and twists of the spine to create perfect "six-pack" abs or to sculpt a narrow waist without realizing that they may be wasting time and energy—never mind that they may also be damaging their low backs.

The link between low-back pain and weak abdominals is finally becoming recognized, and most people who work out now devote at least some of their exercise time to abdominal conditioning. Some even keep records of the number of sit-ups they do on mats or with machines. Why then are so many disappointed with the results? Why is low-back pain or discomfort so common after workouts?

Imagine the spine as a multisegmented flagpole. The long, superficial muscles of the trunk are similar to the guy wires that balance the flagpole. These large muscles, closest to the outside of the body, span greater distances than the deep muscles and allow for larger range-of-motion actions such as arching the back or bending the spine. The small spinal muscles, more internal to the body, support the links between each segment of the pole. These stabilizing muscles, also called core muscles, are the deep muscles of the abdomen and low back that provide stability for the spine. If these deep muscles do not perform effectively the flagpole will become unstable. And most important of all, if these deep muscles do not have the endurance capacity to do their job of supporting the spine, other muscles may be recruited to fill in, performing in ways for which they are not designed.

Old-style methods for abdominal conditioning tend to drill the body in one fixed direction or pattern. But such movements are not very functional: in daily motion our bodies curl forward, extend out, rotate, and bend sideways; our limbs swivel inward and outward, across the midline of the body and away. Traditional exercises strengthen mainly the outer layer of the body—the rectus abdominis, for example, a superficial abdominal muscle that runs vertically down the abdomen. The role of the rectus is to flex the trunk, but this muscle does not directly support the spine in sitting or standing—nor does it directly assist in healing or preventing low-back pain.

Another point of confusion in traditional abs conditioning involves the hip-flexor muscle known as the psoas, a long, strong muscle that originates on the bony parts of the vertebrae of the lower spine, crosses the front of the pelvis, and attaches at the top of the thighbone. This very deep muscle is not usually considered a stabilizing muscle because its role is to connect core to leg, not core to core. It is very strong, however, and can rush to the aid of the abdominals in traditional conditioning exercises. Consider the abs machine that supports your body weight on your forearms and allows your legs to hang freely. As you lift your knees to perform the exercise, the burn you feel is in the hip flexors (including the quadriceps) and in the superficial rectus abdominis muscle, not in the deep abdominals.

The same occurs with standard sit-ups, the number and speed of which is still unfortunately used as a measure of fitness in many sports facilities. Some trainers feel that bending the knees or digging the heels into the mat during sit-ups will disable the psoas, but Stuart McGill, Ph.D., a leading expert on stabilization and low-back disorders, has proved this to be ill founded. He discovered that straight-leg, bent-knee, and heel-on-the-mat sit-ups all involve considerable psoas activation and impose considerable spinal compression. McGill recommends the curl-up over the sit-up. The curl-up is a much smaller movement; keeping the pelvis stable and maintaining the natural curve in the low back, only the upper body is flexed. McGill also favors side-plank or side-bridge exercises over the traditional twisting-of-the-spine exercises for the abdominal obliques. (In side-plank and side-bridge exercises the exerciser is on her side supported by the elbow or hand as she lifts the hips off the mat.) We will learn variations of the side-bridge exercise later in the book.

The basic gist of the above information is this: What results from pinning your feet under a trainer's hands and curling rapidly upward are strong hip flexors, not strong deep abdominals. Many repetitions with rapid speed can compress the low back and aggravate low-back pain. Strong, shortened hip flexors can drag the low back into an arch. Fast crunches can also pull neck muscles and hunch shoulders, causing neck pain.

Learning from the Latest Research

Experts in the field of rehabilitation have known for a while that a strong abdominal core protects the spine, but until recently they were not completely sure as to how this process works. In his highly accessible book, *Spinal Stabilization: The New Science of Back Pain*, Rick Jemmett spells out the crucial role that the deepest abdominal muscle has on the spine. The transversus abdominis attaches through the fascia directly onto the spinal column and is thus able to "stabilize individual vertebrae of the lower back, preventing excess sliding and tilting motions." Jemmett reviews the latest research from Canada, the United States, Japan, and Australia and concludes that various muscles of the spine have different functions. The deepest layer consists of small muscles

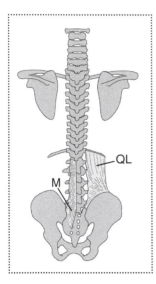

deep back muscles

Stuart McGill, Ph.D., and his associates believe that all of the trunk muscles play some role in stabilization, but multifidus and quadratus lumborum have been identified as key back stabilizers.

One of the deepest of the back extensors, the multifidus muscles consist of small bundles that pass from one vertebra to another. Multifidus have been shown to assist the contraction of the transversus abdominis and vice versa. Quadratus lumborum attaches each vertebra of the low back with the ribs and upper rim of the back of the pelvis. When contracted this muscle causes sidebending of the lumbar spine and rib cage.

of the spine and ligaments that steady the spine and act as "position sensors," supplying the brain with critical information on the position of the joints of the vertebrae. The next layer is the stabilizers—deep muscles of the abdomen (transversus abdominis, internal oblique) and the back (multifidus, quadratus lumborum). Their function is to stabilize the low back and spine and keep them free from pain. Finally, the outer, or superficial, layer consists of large muscles (rectus abdominis, erector spinae, external oblique) that create powerful movements, such as flexing and extending the spine. Movements of the outer layer can be performed safely once the stabilizers provide a strong foundation.

Conventional abdominal- and back-strengthening practices overemphasize the large muscles of the trunk, leaving, as Jemmett writes, "athletes and physio patients physically unprepared for their work or sports activity."

A research team at the University of Queensland, Australia, has garnered a lot of attention lately for its assertion that a person's ability to locate and hold the deep abdominal connection can result in a notable reduction of low-back pain. The researchers—Carolyn Richardson, Gwendolen Jull, Paul Hodges, and Julie Hides—conclude that if the abdominal wall bulges during a movement it is probable that the deep transversus abdominis has stopped functioning and has lost its "corset-like contraction," which enhances stability in the pelvis and low back by increasing the stiffness of the lumbar spine and protecting injured segments of the back if they happen to be present. Stiffness of the lumbar spine during exercise does not mean lack of flexibility in the joints but a spine that has potential for full movement while remaining solid and correctly aligned.

Stuart McGill emphasizes building muscular endurance as the most sound approach to stabilizing the low back. To build endurance in the stabilizers he suggests adding isometric contractions (holding a contraction without moving the body) while working with the abdominals activated, or "braced," and the body in neutral spine. (Neutral spine is a position that maintains the natural curves in the spine without flattening or exaggerating them.) Whether working with rehab patients or high-performance athletes, McGill stresses "sparing the spine" and continually "grooving" healthy motor and movement patterns.

This new research is important for trainers and students alike, as there is much crossover between the rehabilitation and fitness worlds. A clear understanding of how our low back and abdominals work is crucial for anyone designing or participating in an exercise program. As this current information spreads throughout the fitness world, more trainers and instructors are teaching the techniques of "bracing," or "readying," the abs and "moving from the core." However, students and trainers alike must make doubly sure that they are targeting the correct muscles. How can the average person or athlete distinguish between a deep and a superficial muscle? What will they feel if the correct connection is made? And once a deep muscle is located and trained, how can it be integrated into a healthy movement pattern?

The Pilates Powerhouse

During the First World War, German-born Joseph H. Pilates (1880–1967) devised a series of exercises to help people overcome injuries and postural problems. The founder of the now-famous Pilates Method of body conditioning did not have access to the research that we have today, but his theories of movement were well ahead of his time. He regarded the abdominal area, in conjunction with the deep spinal muscles, as the center, or "powerhouse," of the body. He perceived the powerhouse, the "girdle of strength," as the area between the bottom ribs and the pelvis, the region that connects the abdomen with the low back and buttocks. For Pilates, who studied yoga and Zen meditation as well as Western exercise disciplines, this circular belt of supporting abdominal and spinal muscles was a mental and spiritual center as well as a physical, gravitational one.

One of the fundamental principles behind the acclaimed Pilates Method is that the powerhouse is the center of all movement: the stronger the powerhouse, the more powerful and efficient the movement. So before each Pilates exercise one recruits the core by gently pulling in the navel and engaging the deep centering muscles. (See the sidebar "The Core Stablizing Muscles" on page 9.) The goal is to keep the midsection still and stable while precise movements of the arms and legs are executed. It is important, however, to distinguish between movements of everyday life and conscious movements from the powerhouse. We do not want a chronic tight contraction of the abdominals on a moment-by-moment basis in our days, as this interferes with the pump-like downward motion of the diaphragm. Engagement of the core muscles should happen only as part of a workout and fitness regime or before lifting a load, not as a way of life.

The three abdominal muscles—the rectus abdominis, the external and internal obliques, and the transversus abdominis, with the key player being transversus abdominis—work with the spinal muscles (the most important being multifidus and quadratus lumborum) to make up the powerhouse. Pilates practitioners are now also including the pelvic floor in the powerhouse because of the way in which this sling of muscles and ligaments connects through the nervous system to the deep abdominals. Located on the bottom

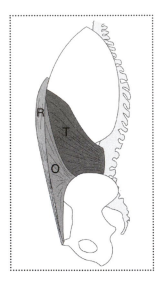

the abdominal muscles

Transversus abdominis is the deepest of the four abdominal muscles. It wraps horizontally around the waist and stabilizes the lumbar spine by narrowing the abdominal wall. This muscle has attracted a lot of attention lately because of its association with the prevention of low-back pain.

Next are the internal and external obliques. These are the natural corset of the body, responsible for sidebending and twisting the spine.

Finally, the long superficial rectus abdominis runs up from the pubic bone to the bottom of the sternum and lower rib cartilages. It is responsible for flexing the trunk, and it does flatten the abdomen.

of the pelvis, the pelvic floor is comprised of the muscles used to control the flow of urine and solid waste from the body. Strengthening the muscles of the pelvic floor is important for men and women and will be discussed further in "Abs on the Ball Fundamentals."

Many in the fitness and rehabilitation worlds believe that working from the powerhouse, or the deep core, is the most effective and safe way to exercise the body. I have seen very favorable results when working with this key principle in mind. This is why I have chosen a Pilates approach to *Abs on the Ball*, even though some of the exercises presented here are not Pilates-based in origin. The Pilates Method is supported by the latest research in rehabilitation and body conditioning and is highly recommended by doctors, physical therapists, and other practitioners around the world.

The Ball As Perfect Partner

Using a Pilates approach is only part of what makes Abs on the Ball so unique. The other element is that you will be using a ball to enhance your workout.

The secret of the ball's success is its most prominent feature—its spherical shape. Unlike any mat or machine, the ball is a mobile surface. The instability of the ball "jump-starts" dormant muscles, recruiting both deep as well as superficial muscle fibers. Paul Chek, an internationally recognized exercise and spine-care specialist, known for his pioneering work in athletic conditioning using exercise balls, explains how the unsteadiness of the ball threatens the reflexes of the body so that the organism starts to fire the stabilizing muscles "out of absolute necessity." Stuart McGill found that a curl-up performed on a ball with the feet on the ground virtually doubled the abdominal-muscle activation of a curl-up performed on a stable surface. The effort of working on a mobile surface creates a much higher demand on the motor system. An exercise with the ball requires complete focus; even as it builds the abdominal core it also trains deep muscles in the back, hips, legs, and arms.

Utilizing the full range of motion is a much more balanced and useful way to work the abdominals. While working on a round surface you will be focusing on stretching out the abdominals, not just shortening them by barreling through a series of swift and vigorous crunches. You will feel how the lengthening (eccentric) contraction is just as important as the "curling up," or shortening (concentric), contraction. In fact, the lengthening contraction, where you use the muscles as brakes as you elongate the body carefully back into its starting position on the ball or mat, is more work for the muscles. In some cases we will hold the body in a position without movement, increasing the tension in the muscle without changing its length. This is called an isometric contraction, and it builds the endurance of the muscles.

The ball will require that you slow down the exercise, giving you time to engage the correct muscles as you pay attention to how the exercises are performed. For some of the exercises we will be using an ultra-soft nine-inch ball called the Overball. This small ball is extremely helpful for keeping the legs in alignment. A gentle squeeze on the small ball engages the inner thighs and aids most people in locating the muscles of the pelvic floor, at the floor of the abdominal area. The small ball is firm enough to add resistance but soft enough to respond to weight changes. We will also use the small ball to suspend the hips off the mat, support the low back in correct posture, and take the pressure off the neck as we tone the abdominals, buttocks, and thighs.

Small or large, the ball will keep your abs enlivened. It will help balance your workout by alternating between upper and lower abdominals and will condition the obliques and quadratus lumborum, the crisscross muscles that shape your waist and allow your spine to rotate and sidebend. We will also work prone, on the belly, in order to train the deep back muscles and on the side to work the muscles that sideflex and rotate. You should find pleasure, not pain, in these unusual and varied exercises designed to build superb abdominal strength and a healthy back. But before you begin, study the fundamentals thoroughly and return to them often in order to understand the exercises and perform them safely and effectively.

2
Abs on the Ball
Fundamentals

The Fundamental Exercises at the beginning of each practice chapter that follows are designed to put into practice the concepts discussed below. As mentioned earlier, for most people—even seasoned athletes—it is necessary first to isolate and train the deep muscles of the back and abdomen before embarking on the more difficult exercises. To do so we use small movements that reprogram the body in a safe and functional way. That is the basis of the Fundamental Exercises. The new awareness and core strength developed through these exercises is then integrated into the basic, intermediate, and advanced Abs on the Ball exercises. Don't skip reading about these key concepts and practicing the Fundamental Exercises at the beginning of each practice chapter.

The Breath: A Crucial Starting Point

We are inhaling through the nose and exhaling through the mouth. On the exhale, make sure the navel is gently pulled in and the abdominals are activated.

We are trying to guide the breath not into the abdominals or the upper chest but into the back of the rib cage. So often students will ask me why we are not breathing into the belly. In daily life we do not want a chronic tight contraction of the abdominals. However, when we start to move from the abdominal center or inner core of support called the powerhouse, we need to make sure that the centering muscles are fully engaged to protect the low back. The breath we are practicing here is rib-cage breathing, or diaphragmatic breathing. The diaphragm is a dome-shaped breathing muscle that assists the stabilizers in supporting the spine. On the inhalation the abdomen may gently rise. However, on the exhalation, make sure the navel is pulled in so that the transversus abdominis and the obliques can tighten around the spine. The out breath should be relaxed and complete, and should aid you in finding the abdominal connection.

There is a breathing pattern to accompany each exercise in this book. These patterns are flexible and can be altered to meet each person's needs. A general rule of thumb is this: Inhale to prepare, scanning the body to check alignment, and exhale on the exertion. Above all, do not force the breath or hold your breath.

The Key Player: Transversus Abdominis

Place your three longest fingers one inch inside your hipbones, press in deeply, and cough. The muscle that you feel is the transversus abdominis. With the correct contraction you will feel a tension in your fingertips as the abdominal wall narrows.

Transversus abdominis is the deepest and most important abdominal muscle. It wraps horizontally around your waist like a corset and stabilizes the low back by narrowing the abdominal wall. Now that you have located the muscle, place your fingers here from time to time as you perform the exercises to make sure the muscle is working. It is a deep muscle: you need to push in deeply enough to feel it. Remember that the abdominal wall narrows when the transversus abdominis is properly engaged. If your fingertips are pushed out, or your abdominals bulge or pop out, then you have lost the deep connection.

The Fundamental Exercises at the beginning of each practice chapter help to isolate and train the transversus abdominis. Keep coming back to these fundamentals and recheck at regular intervals that you have the correct contraction. If you are still having trouble finding the transversus abdominis you may need to work with a qualified physiotherapist or experienced Pilates practitioner trained in rehabilitation to help you identify this muscle for the first time. Don't forget to use your breath to aid you. Once you have located the correct muscle, as often as possible try to maintain the deep contraction before adding movement of the arms and legs.

Connecting Navel to Spine

Use your navel to gently draw your lower belly into your spine. Think of narrowing your waist, not just flattening it. Connecting the navel to the spine protects the spine and hollows the belly by activating the deep abdominal muscles.

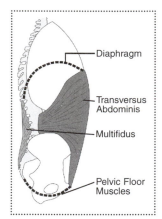

Diaphragm

Transversus Abdominis

Multifidus

Pelvic Floor Muscles

the core stabilizing muscles

The stabilizing, or "core," muscles provide support for the pelvis and low back by increasing the stiffness of the lumbar spine and protecting injured segments of the back if they happen to be present. The Australian authorities on spinal stabilization describe these muscles as a three-dimensional cylinder.

On the front and sides of the cylinder are the deep transversus abdominis; on the back wall are the multifidus. The base of the cylinder is made up by the pelvic floor muscles, and the lid by the diaphragm, a dome-shaped breathing muscle. The stability of the low back depends on the core muscles being strong and working together to transform the abdomen and spine into a rigid cylinder.

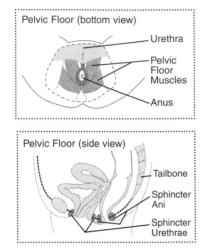

Pelvic Floor (bottom view)

— Urethra

— Pelvic Floor Muscles

— Anus

Pelvic Floor (side view)

— Tailbone

— Sphincter Ani

— Sphincter Urethrae

the pelvic floor muscles

Located on the bottom of the pelvis, the pelvic floor muscles are a sling of muscles and ligaments that suspend from the tailbone and sitz bones to the pubic bone and hold the inner organs within the pelvis. These muscles connect through the nervous system to the deep abdominals.

Tightening the pelvic floor helps men and women find the deep abdominal connection.

"Zip up and hollow," writes Lynne Robinson, the famous Pilates author. "Imagine you are zipping the muscles from the pubic bone up to the navel, as if you were getting into a pair of jeans that are too tight." Her key words here are *from the pubic bone up to the navel*. Think low. Do not simply suck in your gut, because for most people this means hollowing the rib cage and the upper abdominals. Think of gently drawing in your *lower* abdomen, between navel and pubic bone. Narrow your waist rather than just flatten it. Remember, it is the breath—the exhalation—that will aid you in activating the deep abdominals.

The Pelvic Floor: The "Elevator" at the Bottom of the Powerhouse

Contracting the pelvic floor is a sure way for men and women to activate the deep abdominals, because there is a neurological connection between the pelvic floor and the transversus abdominis.

Located on the bottom of the pelvis, the pelvic-floor muscles are engaged when controlling the flow of urine and other waste from the body. This sling of muscles and ligaments connecting tailbone and sitz bones to the pubic bone holds the inner organs within the pelvis. These muscles connect through the nervous system to the deep abdominals. Pelvic floor contractions may be known to some as Kegel exercises, the exercises given to pre- and postnatal women for toning the pelvic floor. Tightening the pelvic floor helps men and women find the deep abdominal connection.

Think of an elevator lifting up and creating support for the entire abdominal area. We will use the large and small ball to learn to power up the pelvic floor elevator and engage the deep muscles of the powerhouse.

Neutral Pelvis

Neutral pelvis is a stance that maintains the natural curve in the low back and places the pelvis in the safest and least stressful position.

Lying on your back on the mat, try slipping a hand under your low back. With most body shapes you should be able to ease your fingers into the space between the mat and your back. It is desirable that this space be smaller rather than gaping. Some people may need to tilt the pelvis slightly upward until they are able to isolate and control the abdominals to maintain neutral pelvis.

In the practice section of the book we will learn how to consistently find neutral pelvis and then how to maintain it while adding movement. Why are we so interested in the natural curve of the low back? Neutral pelvis places the pelvis in its best shock-absorbing position and helps facilitate the deep contraction of the waist-narrowing transversus abdominis. When lying on your back in neutral pelvis the two hipbones and the pubic bone are in the same plane. The exact curvature of neutral pelvis may vary from person to person.

One way to find neutral spine is to sit on the ball and bounce three times. The body will usually react by lengthening into optimal posture. Do not flatten the low-back curve or exaggerate it when sitting on the ball or lying on the mat. We simply want to work with the natural curve.

There is one exception to neutral pelvis position, an exception endorsed by most Pilates practitioners. It may be desirable when lying on the mat and extending the legs into the air for the low back to flatten on the mat. In some advanced abdominal work it may be hazardous to the low back if the low back is not anchored securely on the mat and is instead allowed to arch up as the abdominals bulge out. In either case, do not force the low back downward so that the buttocks or the hips tense up. As the low back lengthens downward the sacrum—the five fused vertebrae at the base of the spine—should always remain in contact with the mat, and the buttocks should not lift.

Inside Out

Train the inside muscles first, then train the outer layer.

We aim to work from the inside out. The superficial rectus abdominis and the large outer muscles of the trunk, such as erector spinae, are similar to the guy wires that balance a flagpole Yet it is the deep muscles that provide support in the links between each segment of the spine. The stronger the small, deep muscles are, the more forcefully the large, superficial muscles can work. If the deep-muscle system does not supply inner support for outer muscles, the larger superficial muscles may be targeted to take over and perform in ways for which they are not designed.

Everyday Abs

Abdominal and low-back strength is essential for everyday life, sports, and recreational activities.

This work should not stop when you roll off your ball. Learn to stabilize the powerhouse properly in all your daily activities to prevent injury. Whether you are digging in the garden, hoisting a heavy object overhead, or lifting a child from the ground, it is the strength of the deep centering muscles of the abdomen and back that enable you to perform the movements safely. Draw the navel gently into the spine and initiate your movement from the powerhouse. If you have recurring low-back pain see a physiotherapist knowledgeable in the mechanics of deep abdominal training.

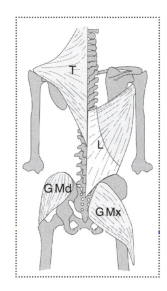

the prime movers

Latissimus dorsi is a large muscle that originates on the low back and mid-back, wraps around the trunk, and fastens onto the upper arms. Trapezius, another superficial back muscle, is a long diamond-shaped muscle spanning the neck and upper and midback. The gluteals are the powerful muscles of the buttocks.

These large muscles, sometimes called prime movers, are designed for forceful actions of brief duration. Movements of the outer layer should only be added once the deep stabilizers provide a strong foundation for those movements. The stronger the small, deep muscles, the more forcefully the large, superficial muscles will work to help you kick, leap, and throw.

Quality, Not Quantity

Pushing the body too far too fast encourages the wrong muscles and creates incorrect movement patterns.

This final concept is perhaps the most important of all. Many of us are not used to training the invisible, inner-layer muscles. Old-style and more familiar methods focus on strengthening the more visible outer muscles of the torso, such as the latissimus dorsi, the trapezius, and the gluteals, to name a few. These large muscles are sometimes called *prime movers*. Training of the outer layer can be added to a fitness program once the deep stabilizers have been conditioned to provide strong support. We have to reprogram the body and the mind to this new approach. Start with few repetitions at low intensity. Pushing the body too far too fast simply encourages the wrong muscles to work and creates incorrect patterns of movement.

Quality, not quantity, is the refrain of Abs on the Ball work. We desire a quality of movement that is controlled and precise. This may be a drastically different approach to your usual workout. You may also be surprised to see a recommendation of only eight or less repetitions per exercise. Ideally, we do not stop between the exercises. Instead move directly from one exercise to the next, with good technique, so that endurance can be built.

3
Final Points

No matter what your level of fitness, start your practice of this new approach to abdominal training with chapter 4, "Basic Abs on the Ball." When the inner system is strong, accomplished athletes and serious gym buffs will be amazed at how much more adept they are with jumps, kicks, or weight lifting. The exercises have been organized to keep the sequence of movement flowing and to promote a balanced development of muscles that flex, extend, side-flex, and rotate. Don't skip the fundamentals at the opening of each practice chapter. They are very effective exercises in themselves and will help you identify, isolate, and strengthen the proper muscles, as well as align your body correctly.

As you are learning these exercises keep to the order in which they are presented, even if you only do a few at a time. If you are out of shape or recovering from an injury you will have to *gradually* increase the number of exercises you practice, being careful to maintain good technique. People who are recovering from an injury may need to begin rehabilitation on a stable surface instead of a ball. See your medical practitioner to make sure these exercises are for you. If you are an intermediate student and are suddenly injured or develop neck strain or low-back pain, use the basic Abs on the Ball exercises (chapter 4) to keep your body moving despite your physical constraints.

Start with one exercise at a time. Read through all the instructions before you begin and pay attention to the watchpoints and modifications. Perseverance pays off. Slow things down; visualize what you are trying to accomplish

our navel, our center

When I first told people I was writing a new book called *Abs on the Ball*, I was reminded that for many our abdomens are an emotionally charged part of the body, a barometer of strength and vulnerability. One man, hiding behind a deep laugh that made his own belly quiver, joked about being "ruled by his stomach." A woman spoke about her pitch-perfect intuition, inherited from her grandmother, allowing her to discern a situation "from her guts." Even pronouncing the word *abs* caused people to physically adjust their bodies, shift forward in their chairs, or stand taller.

with each move. A small percentage of students experience motion sickness when using the ball. If you feel the onset of motion sickness, stop and take some deep breaths. Immediately make note of which exercise brought on the sensation. Make this exercise a much smaller movement or omit it completely. Those who suffer from vertigo should restrict themselves to ballwork on the mat and should seek advice from their doctors.

Working on a mobile ball will tax you in new ways. The nervous system is provoked much more on a ball than on a mat; neuromuscular fatigue sets in quickly and coordination breaks down. Because of this, the more challenging exercises should only be added one or two at a time near the beginning, not at the end, of a workout, *but only after you have warmed up*. Warming the body is accomplished by engaging in a gentle activity that actually heats the muscles. (Stretching should never be used as a strategy for warming the body; it is important to warm up *before* you stretch.) Prior to practicing Abs on the Ball exercises make sure you do some gentle aerobic moves to raise your heart rate, or take a ten-minute walk. You might also practice the Fifteen-minute Basic Abs Workout (see page 162) as a way to warm up the body.

Once you are warmed up, add challenging variations to an exercise only when you are able to maintain optimal form with easier versions. I repeat: Do not push yourself too far too fast. As fatigue sets in, seasoned athletes as well as beginners resort to the overdeveloped strength of the outside layer of muscles, which is exactly what we do not want.

The Right Ball for You

When people of all ages and any level of fitness see a ball they are eager to begin to play or exercise. But before you do so please consider some general guidelines. Following these hints and precautions could make the difference between a safe and competent workout and a clumsy, ineffectual, and even risky one.

Exercise balls are inexpensive and widely available in health and fitness shops. Be warned: All balls are not created equal. Some are cheap to the touch and to the smell. I personally prefer Fitballs (see page 189 for ordering information). I use only Fitballs in my teaching and for my personal workouts because they have an excellent surface that is not dangerously slippery but is pliable and firm without being heavy. Most important of all, they are burst resistant. If you accidentally roll over a small rock or tack they will not explode—they will deflate gradually. Fitballs even have a faint pleasant vanilla aroma, not a strong vinyl smell. They are latex-free and weight-tested to 1,000 pounds (455 kilograms) for normal use.

The appropriate size of the ball is a subject of debate among teachers and depends on the exercise method you will be using. In Abs on the Ball we are not bouncing on the ball, so I find the 55-cm ball is perfect unless you are very tall. The larger the ball, the heavier and more unwieldy it is. As a general rule, when sitting on the ball the hips and knees should be bent at as close to a 90-degree angle as possible. This usually translates to a 55-cm ball for people 5' to 5'8", and a 65-cm ball for people measuring 5'8" to 6'2".

The small ball shown in the book is a nine-inch Overball. Like the Fitball, it is manufactured in the Ledraplastic factory in Italy. The Overball has a sensual, skinlike, pliable surface that compresses easily and will not hurt if the ball is thrown or bruise your body if it is squeezed. The Overball is an ultralight, inexpensive, must-have second ball that can be used in place of the Pilates circle or small barrel to support or stretch the body and help locate muscles. Overballs are weight-tested to 440 pounds (200 kilograms) and are inflated with a straw. (See page 189 for ordering information.) A chi ball, a soft child's ball called a Gertie ball, or a large square or round piece of foam will work just as well.

FIRM VERSUS SOGGY

Air pressure in the ball should be greater for heavier students than for lighter ones. I personally prefer a slightly soggy, or underinflated, small or large ball for most of this work. A slightly deflated ball is more responsive to the body. As well as being comfortable, it will not compress the chest and breasts or dig into the pelvic area. Mari Naumovski, creator of BodySpheres ballwork, uses the analogy drawn from a dance form called contact improvisation to discuss the ball's firmness. She explains that when one is dancing with a partner who is very muscle bound—a description analogous to a highly inflated ball—it can be difficult to feel movement travel through the different layers of the body.

A slightly softer ball is also easier for beginners, because it provides a larger base of support. For some of the more demanding exercises, however, a firm ball gives better support for completing an exercise properly. If you are doing a lot of sitting or bouncing on the ball then a firm ball, sized correctly, is desirable.

Balls are blown up according to diameter (height off the floor), not air pressure. A yardstick will help you inflate to the maximum diameter, which is printed on the ball and on the box in which the ball is sold. Inflate only to the recommended diameter, not bigger. Fitballs come with long plugs that are easy to pull out of the ball to deflate it for travel. Most people find that a bicycle

pregnancy and abdominal exercises

Because of the focus on the abdominal connection and compression of the abdominal wall, many of the exercises in this book are not suitable for pregnant women. Unless very experienced in the Pilates Method, pregnant women should work out in prenatal classes with exercises carefully designed for each trimester.

After giving birth, and receiving clearance from your health care practitioner, you will find Abs on the Ball exercises excellent for strengthening the pelvic floor and the abdominals. Weak abdominals can leave a new mother prone to back injury, so start as soon as your doctor, midwife, or nurse practitioner allows you.

If you give birth by cesarean section you will need to wait at least six weeks to begin Abs on the Ball exercises, and because the cesarean process involves cutting through the abdominal muscles, it may take many months to feel your abdominals again. Start with the fundamentals and work slowly through the basic exercises after consulting with your doctor or health care practitioner.

pump is simply not forceful enough for inflating the larger balls. Use an air raft or mattress pump or go to a gas station and use a cone-shaped trigger nozzle. I use a small inexpensive plastic pump that is totally portable and very effective for inflating the ball. (See page 189 for ordering information.)

SMALL VERSUS LARGE

Working with a small ball is not necessarily easier than working with a large one. Some students prefer the small ball because it is possible to work very precisely, you are able to target muscles on a different level, and the student and teacher alike can see the body clearly to discern pelvis and body placement. The small ball has definite portability and storage advantages, and I have found a meditative and sensuous quality when working with it as it responds more readily to weight changes and breath. Some exercises, however, can only be performed with the large ball. The large ball is able to lift the body up into the air and creates more resistance and more opportunities for increasing range of movement. The sense of accomplishment is high when skillfully maneuvering on a large ball. Some exercises can be performed with either the small or large ball, though some moves are particularly designed for one ball or the other.

Helpful Hints and Precautions

Check with your doctor or health care practitioner to make sure these exercises are suitable for you. Pay attention to modifications and stop if there is any discomfort. If in doubt, avoid an exercise. If you are pregnant see the sidebar on this page.

In addition to these general suggestions, here are some other points to keep in mind as you begin your practice.

- "Less is more." If you are experiencing pain, you are pushing yourself too hard.
- With any exercise routine it is not advisable to exercise after a meal. This is especially so with Abs on the Ball.
- Start gradually. Make sure you have drinking water at hand.
- Bare feet connect best with the ground. If you still find your feet slipping, use rubber-soled shoes or sneakers.
- Work on a slip-resistant yoga mat or a nonslip rug.
- Make sure you have plenty of space around you.
- Avoid loose clothing and tie back long hair as they can get caught under the ball.

- Check that the area is clear of staples, tacks, or any other sharp objects that may damage the ball. Inspect the ball each time before you use it. This is especially important in a gym setting where floors may be dirty and exercise balls may have been tossed against sharp pieces of equipment.
- Inflate balls at room temperature. Do not inflate at hot or cold temperatures.
- Keep the balls clean. A dirty exercise ball is unhygienic and can be slippery. Most balls clean up quickly with a cloth and, if necessary, a bit of soapy water.
- Make sure that the ball you are working on is burst resistant. There are many cheap balls on the market today that do not have this important safety feature.
- Do not use the balls outside and do not let animals play with the balls. Children should never be left unattended with a ball that is too large for them.
- Keep your ball out of direct sunlight and away from direct heat sources. Do not leave a ball fully inflated inside a hot car.
- Do not attempt to repair a damaged ball. Get rid of it.

One Final Word

At the back of the book you will find fifteen- and thirty-minute basic, intermediate, and advanced abdominal workouts. For strong abdominals and the health of the low back, try to do one of these workouts every day or every second day. The body, however, cannot live on abdominal exercises alone. Include cardiovascular and strength training in your workouts. Flexibility is also important for back health: strong yet flexible muscles are better able to meet everyday and sports activities without injury and strain. For more information on cardiovascular, strength training, or stretching using a ball please refer to the books and videos listed on the resources page. Again, check with your doctor or health care practitioner before starting this or any other exercise program.

4

Basic Abs on the Ball

The exercises in this chapter are a great starting point for everyone, no matter what your level of fitness or prior training. The gentle yet effective exercises here are designed to increase the endurance of the abdominal, inner thigh, buttock, and back muscles and, in some cases, alleviate moderate low-back pain.

Pay particular attention to the Fundamental Exercises. They will teach you neutral pelvis and head positions as well as how to isolate and train the deep transversus abdominis and pelvic floor muscles. In some ways the fundamentals are the hardest exercises of all not in terms of physical strength, but because such small, precise movements are very challenging for many people. Persevere and repeat them often.

As you move from the fundamentals into the basic exercises take care not to push yourself too far too fast. Maintain the body in good alignment and think of the deep centering muscles working together to protect the spine and keep the pelvis stable. If you have a sore neck leave your head on the mat or place your hands behind your neck to support it whenever you lift your head off the mat. Keep your shoulders relaxed downward instead of lifted toward your ears in order to avoid neck tension. Make sure you are initiating each move with breath, and use the breath to move the body as efficiently as possible.

Practicing the Fundamentals

The Fundamental Exercises are small, precise programming exercises designed to practice proper breathing, review body placement, and locate the proper muscles before you begin the basic exercises. "Neutral pelvis," "pelvic floor," "navel-to-spine connection"—you are learning a new language, and these five fundamentals will prime your body, and your mind, for this new experience. Work slowly and methodically through all five Fundamental Exercises until you are satisfied that your body understands these important concepts. Then you will be ready to move on to the Basic Exercises.

Fundamental #1: Back Breathing

Diaphragmatic breathing is crucial to the Abs on the Ball exercises. The diaphragm is a dome-shaped muscular wall between the chest and the abdominals. It is designed to work like a pump: on the in breath it contracts and moves downward, drawing in air. On the out breath the diaphragm relaxes and the dome rises, discharging used air. In this exercise try to guide the air into the lower rib cage and back, not into the abdominals or upper chest. Directing the air into the lower rib cage and the back assures that the diaphragm is at work in your breathing. Remember, there is evidence that the diaphragm assists the other stabilizers to provide spinal support. (See the sidebar "The Core Stabilizing Muscles" on page 9.) For Side Breathing use a soggy ball. Direct the breath into the side rib cage and enjoy how the ball responds to the breath. Persevere but don't force the breath.

Purpose To practice diaphragmatic breathing. To direct the breath into the back and side of the rib cage.

Watchpoints • Inhale through the nose; exhale through the mouth with a relaxed jaw. • Focus on the breath and try not to create tension in any part of the body. • If you experience neck or arm strain in Side Breathing, support your head with your hand or drop the head and chest onto the ball.

purpose of the fundamentals

- To practice correct breathing.
- To find your neutral pelvis.
- To learn how to safely lift the head off the mat.
- To activate your pelvic floor, the "elevator" at the bottom of the powerhouse.
- To learn how to isolate and contract the deep abdominal muscles.
- To foster a good working relationship among deep muscles of the abdomen and the low back, the pelvis, and the diaphragm before progressing on to more difficult exercises.

starting position

Lie on your back with your knees bent and your feet hip-distance apart. Wrap your hands around your lower rib cage (fig. 4.1).

movement 1: back breathing

1. Inhale through the nose to expand the rib cage sideways. Exhale through the mouth and imagine the ribs sliding together.

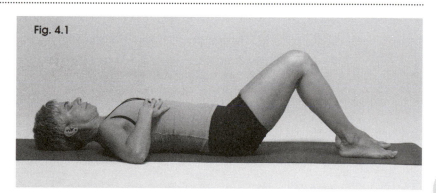

Fig. 4.1

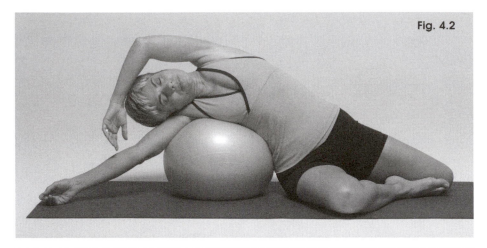

Fig. 4.2

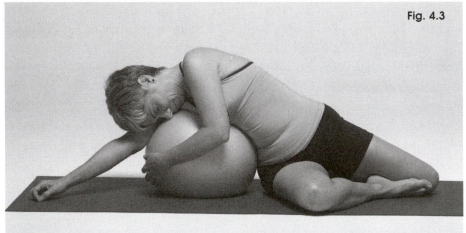

Fig. 4.3

2. Take five more of these deep breaths into the rib cage.

3. Roll over onto your right side and slowly sit up using your arms to help you. Let your head be the last to come up.

movement 2: side breathing

1. Sit with your right side beside your ball. Bend the right knee in front and curl the left foot behind you. Shift your weight onto the right side and allow the right side of the body to relax over the ball, left arm relaxing overhead. Your head can rest on the right shoulder (fig. 4.2).

2. Inhale through the nose to expand the left rib cage.

3. Exhale through the mouth to release.

4. Take five more breaths.

5. Repeat on the left side. Relax your head onto the ball if desired (fig. 4.3).

Fundamental #2: Neutral Pelvis Lying on the Mat

Neutral pelvis is a position that maintains the natural curve in your low back. It puts your spine into optimal relationship with your pelvis and stabilizes the back so that the disks are in a safe, uncompressed position. Lie on your back on the mat. The two hipbones on the front of your pelvis should be parallel with the pubic bone. Slip a hand under your low back—you should be able to ease your fingers into the space between your body and the mat. It is desirable that the space be smaller rather than gaping. This exercise shows how to find neutral pelvis by using the abdominals to tilt the pelvis to feel first too much curve in the low back and then too little. Somewhere between these two extremes is neutral.

Purpose To mobilize the low back and locate neutral pelvis.

Watchpoints • Try not to create tension in any other part of the body. Neither the buttocks nor the thigh muscles should be working in this exercise. Relax them. • Remember to inhale into the back ribs, not the abdomen.

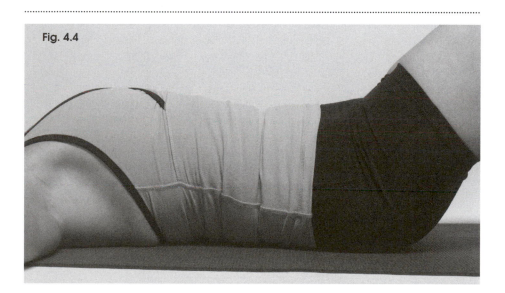

Fig. 4.4

starting position

Lie on your back with your knees bent. Feet should be hip-distance apart and parallel, in line with your knees; knees are in line with your hips.

movement: tilting the pelvis in and out of neutral

1. Inhale. Exhale to gently pull the muscles of the low abdomen in, slightly tilting the pelvis and flattening the low back against the mat. The pubic bone will lift (fig. 4.4).

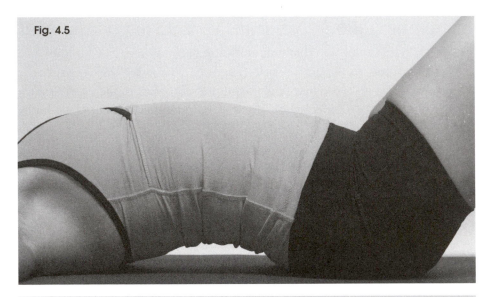

Fig. 4.5

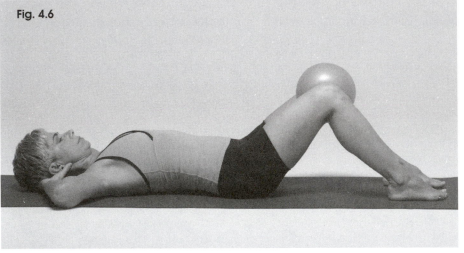

Fig. 4.6

2. Inhale to drop your pubic bone downward so that there is a slope running from the hipbones on the front of your pelvis to your pubic bone. You will feel an exaggerated arch in your back (fig. 4.5).

3. Exhale to use the abdominals to flatten the low back against the mat as you slightly lift your pubic bone, as in the first movement.

4. Repeat several times, tilting the pelvis in both directions.

5. Finish by allowing the pelvis to rest in neutral (fig. 4.6). The tailbone should feel heavy as it lengthens on the mat. Your pelvis is neither tipped up nor dropped. Your hipbones and pubic bone are parallel.

Fundamental #3:
Lifting the Head off the Mat

Many abdominal exercise are performed with the head lifted off the mat. The aim of this exercise is to train the body to lift the heavy head without straining the neck or aggravating neck tension. When practicing this exercise keep three points in mind. First, make sure when lying on your back that your head is not tilted so far back that your neck arches. Drop or nod the chin gently forward as if you want to hold a tennis ball at the throat. In some cases the head may need to rest on a flat pillow to achieve this angle. Second, make sure the shoulders are stabilized and are not raised toward the ears. Keep them in position as you lift the head. Finally, when you do lift the head do so immediately, not as an afterthought. While you may want to place your hands lightly on the base of the skull to help guide your head, use your abdominals—not your hands—to actually lift the head. When the head is lifted your gaze should be on your knees and not on the ceiling.

Purpose To practice lifting the head off the mat safely.

Watchpoints • Move the neck gently and effortlessly. • Do not jam the chin into the chest or poke it into the air. Remember the image of holding a tennis ball between the chin and the chest.

starting position

Lie on your back with your knees bent. Feet should be hip-distance apart and parallel, in line with your knees; knees should be in line with your hips.

movement 1: chin nods

1. Inhale to raise the chin slightly (fig. 4.7).
2. Exhale to drop the chin gently forward as if to hold a tennis ball at the throat. This correction will produce a sensation of lengthening through the neck, which is desirable when the head is resting on the mat.

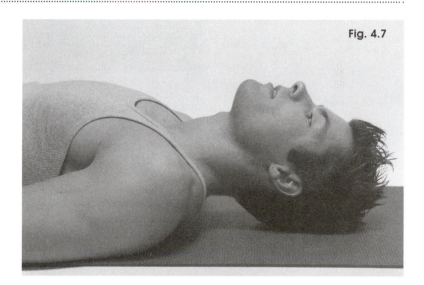

Fig. 4.7

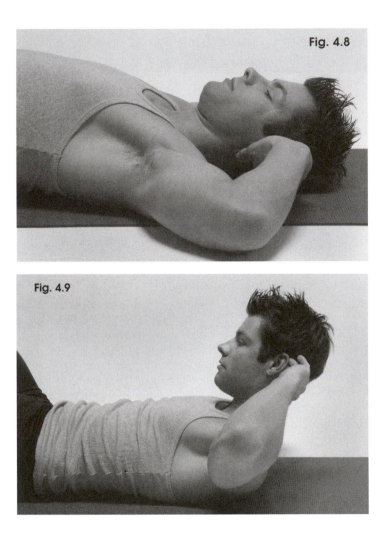

Fig. 4.8

Fig. 4.9

3. Inhale to roll the head back slightly.
4. Exhale to nod the chin.
5. Repeat six times.

movement 2: lifting the head off the mat

1. To avoid pulling on the back of the neck, place your fingertips lightly on the base of the skull behind your ears. Inhale to prepare (fig. 4.8).
2. Exhale to nod the chin and curl the head upward, gently supporting the weight of the head with the hands but using the abdominals to lift the head. Your head should lift immediately. Let your gaze rest on your knees, not on the ceiling (fig. 4.9).
3. Inhale to return the head to the mat.
4. Exhale to nod the chin and curl upward.
5. Repeat six times.

Fundamental #4: Connecting Navel to Spine

Kneeling on all fours is a very effective position for feeling the action of drawing the lower abdominals up and in. The rest of the body—especially the buttocks muscles—are not involved in this action. When learning this subtle contraction take care not to allow any movement in the spine or pelvis. The contraction should be very small and precise. I repeat: this is a minuscule movement. Once you have felt the contraction, maximize its effectiveness by keeping the abdominals connected. This means to hold the deep contraction by continuing to draw the navel inward—pull the area between the navel and pubic bone away from the edge of your pants. Try not to let the tension out of the muscle. You will find that as you keep the deep muscle activated for ten seconds or longer you become even more aware of it, and it will get strong. Then perform the same exercise on a large ball. Use a soggy large ball: it will not compress your chest and it will respond to your body and your breath. Finally, maintain the contraction of the deep abdominals while adding movement of the limbs: in this case, simple hand lifts.

Purpose To learn how to create a strong center by gently drawing in the navel.

Watchpoints • This movement is subtle. The contraction of the abdominals is performed in a slow, controlled manner. Think of drawing in the area between pubic bone and navel. • The buttocks muscles are not involved. Avoid arching or rounding the back or moving the pelvis. • Keep shoulders easing down the back. • Remember to inhale through the nose and exhale through the mouth. Think of sending the breath into the back of the rib cage.

starting position

Start on all fours, taking care to make sure your hands are aligned below the shoulders and your knees are aligned below the hip joints. Weight is equally distributed on all four limbs; knees are apart. Lengthen through the back of the neck so that the gaze is on the mat. The spine is in neutral, not arched or too flat. Elbows are soft, not locked.

movement 1: the contraction

1. Let your belly gently release with gravity without moving the spine or pelvis (fig. 4.10).

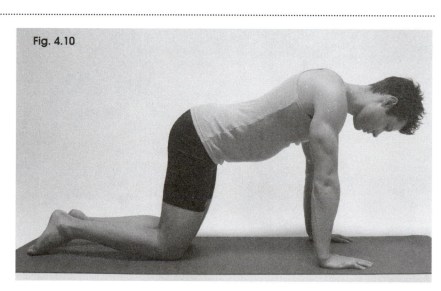

Fig. 4.10

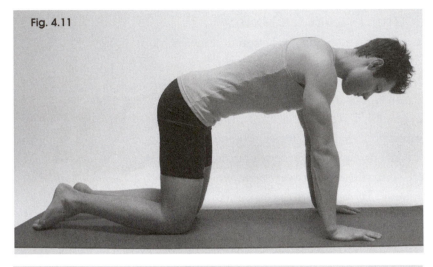

Fig. 4.11

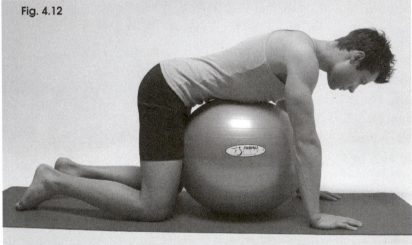

Fig. 4.12

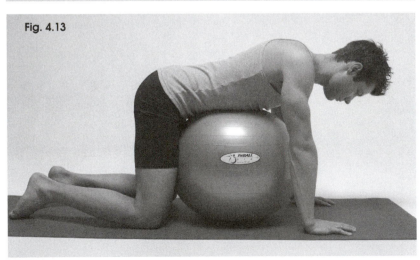

Fig. 4.13

2. Take a couple of easy breaths in and out. Then pull the navel and lower abdomen up and in. Think of drawing in the area between the pubic bone and the navel (fig. 4.11).
3. Inhale and release the navel.
4. Exhale to lift the navel into the spine.
5. Repeat six to eight times.

movement 2: hold contraction

1. Take a couple of easy breaths in and out and then gently pull in the navel and lower abdomen. Think of drawing in the area between the pubic bone and the navel (fig. 4.11).
2. Keep breathing as you hold the contraction for ten seconds. Do not hold your breath.
3. Relax your belly, take a few breaths, and try again, holding the contraction for 15 to 20 seconds. Keep the tension in the deep muscle.
4. Repeat three times.

movement 3: with large ball

1. Lie over a soggy large ball. Hands are directly beneath the shoulders, knees beneath the hips. Depending on the size of the ball you may have your weight on your toes rather than your knees.
2. Inhale to lengthen through the spine.
3. Exhale to lift your navel (fig. 4.12).
4. Inhale to release your navel onto the ball (fig. 4.13).
5. Repeat this movement five times.

movement 4: add hand lifts and contraction

1. Inhale to lengthen through the spine.
2. Exhale to scoop your navel and lift one hand a few inches off the mat (fig. 4.14).
3. Inhale to maintain the contraction as you lower the hand.

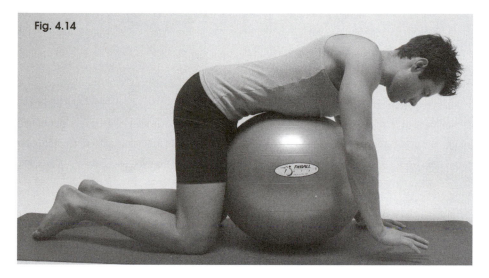

Fig. 4.14

4. Exhale to lift the other hand a few inches off the ground. Keep the abdominals connected. (Try not to let the tension out of the muscle.)

5. Inhale to lower the hand. Exhale to lift the hand.

6. Repeat four times for each side, keeping the abdominals connected for both the in breath and the out breath.

Who Was Joseph Pilates?

German-born Joseph H. Pilates (1880–1967) was an accomplished boxer, gymnast, and circus performer. He personally triumphed over a succession of physical ailments, including asthma and rheumatic fever, by devoting himself to the practice of athletics. Interned in English camps for German nationals during World War I, he began to train other prisoners in his matwork exercises. He also devised makeshift exercise aids with bedsprings or chairs so that people recovering from injuries could exercise safely. Modern versions of these pieces of equipment are found in Pilates studios today.

In the late 1920s Joseph Pilates immigrated to New York and opened a studio. His work attracted many dancers, boxers, and other athletes. Dancers Martha Graham and George Balanchine were among Joseph Pilates' early students.

Originally calling his unique mind/body workout

"Contrology," Pilates fused the best aspects of the Eastern and Western exercise disciplines. From the East he adopted the philosophies of mind/body connection, relaxation, and the importance of flexibility; from the West an emphasis on muscle tone and strength, endurance, and intensity of movement.

The Pilates Method as it is practiced today is a complete and thorough program of mental and physical conditioning. Many of the small therapeutic movements can be modified for people recovering from injuries or intensified to enhance the skill base of elite athletes and dancers. Attracting people of all ages and levels of fitness, the Pilates Method of exercise has become extremely popular worldwide. Its benefits include correcting muscular imbalances, realigning the body, and building core strength from within.

Fundamental #5: Pelvic Floor Exercise

Return to lying on your back but place the small ball between your knees, pelvis in neutral. The goal in movement 1 is to feel how a small squeeze of the inner thighs assists the muscles of the pelvic floor. Without allowing the tailbone to lift off the mat you should feel the anal sphincter and the pelvic floor muscles gently squeeze together as the "elevator" at the bottom of the pelvis draws up. Imagine you have an extremely full bladder and are tightening these muscles to stop the flow of urine while you search for a bathroom. Women may recognize this movement as a Kegel exercise. However, locating the pelvic floor is as important for men as it is for women. Once you have found the correct muscles, the action in movement 2 strengthens the pelvic floor by holding the contraction for five to ten seconds. Remember, the pelvis itself will not move in this exercise: only the muscles draw up and in as they tighten. Notice how the pelvic floor muscles relax during the in breath and tighten during the out breath.

Finally, after isolating the muscles of the pelvic floor place your thumb or three longest fingers one inch in from the hipbones and press inward. The pelvic floor connects through the nervous system to the deep abdominals, so you should feel by the tension on your fingertips that the deep transversus abdominis are also at work.

Purpose To locate the muscles of the pelvic floor and to feel how the pelvic floor contraction triggers the deep abdominals.

Watchpoints • Do not let the pelvis move or tilt. • Remember the inner thigh squeeze is a gentle one. • Keep the tailbone in contact with the mat. Buttocks should be relaxed with no tension in the thighs. • Do not hold your breath in movements 2 and 3.

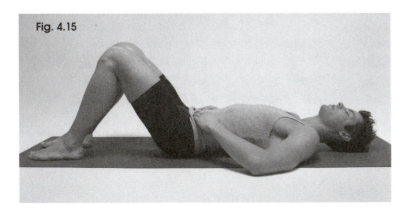
Fig. 4.15

starting position

Lie on your back with your knees bent. Feet should be hip-distance apart and parallel. The small ball is between your knees.

movement 1: finding the pelvic floor

1. Inhale to prepare.
2. Exhale to squeeze the ball slightly, imagining the pelvic floor slowly and gently drawing upward and tightening (fig. 4.15).
3. Inhale to release.
4. Exhale to squeeze the ball slightly.
5. Repeat six times.

movement 2: pelvic floor elevator exercise

1. Inhale. Exhale to gently squeeze the small ball, imagining the pelvic floor slowly drawing upward and tightening. Imagine an elevator ascending from the basement to the first floor.
2. Maintain the elevator on the first floor and hold the contraction for 5 to 10 seconds, breathing naturally.
3. Inhale and exhale to slowly draw the elevator from the first to the second floor. Hold the contraction for 5 to 10 seconds, breathing naturally.
4. Inhale and exhale to slowly draw the elevator from the second to the third floor. Hold the contraction for 5 to 10 seconds, breathing naturally.
5. Release, allowing the elevator to slowly descend to the basment.
6. Repeat the entire sequence once more.

movement 3: feel the transversus abdominis

1. Place your thumb or three largest fingers one inch in from your hipbones and press inward. Inhale.
2. Exhale and tighten the pelvic floor muscles. Maintain this contraction as you draw in the navel and lower abdomen.
3. Can you feel the pressure on your fingertips as the pelvic floor contraction activates the transversus abdominis?
4. Release and repeat four times. Do not hold your breath.

Pelvic Floor Muscles and Stress Incontinence

The pelvic floor muscles hang like a hammock, extending from the pubic bone to the tailbone under the abdominals. To be in good shape these muscles need to be able hold in urine, gas, and feces. These same muscles need to be able to relax as well. A strong pelvic floor is as important for men as for women, because the pelvic floor muscles support the internal organs. A deficiency in these muscles can cause urinary problems in middle age.

Stress incontinence occurs when pressure within the abdomen causes urine to leak out involuntarily during coughing, laughing, or exertion. According to physiotherapist and urge incontinence expert Beate Carrière, stress or urge incontinence affects one in ten men, one in four women, and 17 percent of children between the ages of five and fifteen.

Dr. Arnold Kegel was one of the first authorities to specifically prescribe exercises for the pelvic floor, mainly to women whose pelvic floor muscles were slack from childbirth. "Kegel exercises" were developed in the 1940s; women were instructed to draw the pelvic floor up and in, and to exercise three times a day for twenty minutes. The effectiveness of the exercises depended on motivation and how well the exercises were explained.

More recently, exercise balls have been used with great success in treating stress and urge incontinence and in rehabilitating patients with pelvic floor dysfunction following pregnancy and other conditions. Carrière believes that 90 percent of cases can be greatly improved or cured with simple exercises. She uses firm exercise balls and diaphragmatic breathing to help her patients retrain weak pelvic floor and sphincter muscles, both for prevention and restoration. Movements on the ball, especially in a sitting position, simultaneously and functionally retrain muscles of the pelvic floor, abdomen, and inner thighs. Bouncing on balls can be used as a means for strengthening the pelvic floor as well as testing for deficiencies. Lying on a mat or a bed and gently squeezing a ball or a pillow helps more muscle fibers to be recruited than in an ordinary mat exercise. For some exercises Carrière advocates holding the contraction for 5 to 10 seconds, followed by a rest period of 10 to 15 seconds.

For more information on these exercises see Beate Carrière's video and book, *Exercises for the Pelvic Floor*, listed on the resources page.

The Basic Abs on the Ball Exercises

Once you have completed all five Fundamental Exercises and have a clear picture of the pelvic floor and transversus working first in isolation and then together, you are ready to progress to the Basic Exercises.

Ab Curls with Small Ball

A soft small ball is an excellent tool to help you keep the legs in alignment and make sure the deep *and* the superficial abdominal muscles are working. As the inner thigh, deep abdominal, and pelvic floor muscles work together, the small ball between your knees helps facilitate the contraction of all three. Focus on keeping the ball in place with a gentle squeeze as you contract the abdominals in a slow, controlled manner. Use the exhalation to sink the navel toward the spine. Pause for three seconds at the top of movement 2 to tighten the abdominals before lowering the head to the mat. Watch for bulging abdominals—a sure sign that the deep abdominal connection is lost. From time to time as you perform the exercises, place your hand just inside your hip-bones and press. You will feel pressure on your fingertips as the deep abdominal muscle works. Remember to keep your pelvis in neutral as you curl it upward. Do not lift the tailbone; keep the tailbone heavy on the mat.

Purpose To strengthen the abdominals and flatten the abdomen.

Watchpoints • The pelvis stays in neutral and the tailbone does not lift as you lift the upper body. • Do not curl up too high; the shoulder blades are barely off the mat. • Make sure the head comes up immediately, the gaze on your knees, not the ceiling. • Do not pull on the neck; place hands lightly behind the ears.

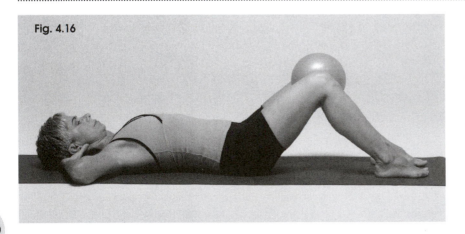

Fig. 4.16

starting position

Lie on your back with your knees bent, feet hip-distance apart and parallel. Hands are loosely clasped behind the ears. Place the small ball between your knees (fig. 4.16).

movement 1: ab curls

1. Inhale to prepare, keeping your head on the mat.
2. Exhale to sink the navel toward the spine and lift the

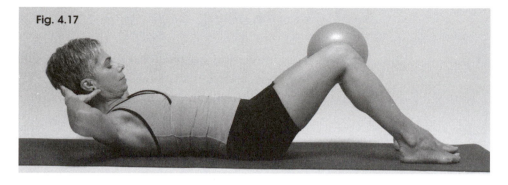

Fig. 4.17

head, flexing the upper body (fig. 4.17).

3. Inhale and stay in this position. Keep the abdominals connected. Imagine you are pulling your navel away from the edge of your pants. Try not to let the tension out of the muscle. Your gaze is on your knees, not on the ceiling.

4. Exhale to return your head to the mat.

5. Repeat eight times, slow and controlled.

movement 2: hold contraction

1. Inhale to prepare with head on the mat.

2. Exhale to sink the navel toward the spine and lift the head, flexing the upper body.

3. Inhale and stay for 3 seconds, tightening your abs. Your gaze is on your knees, not at the ceiling (fig. 4.17).

4. Exhale to return your head to the mat.

5. Repeat four times, slow and controlled.

Incorrect Positions and Poor Form

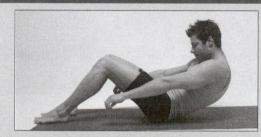

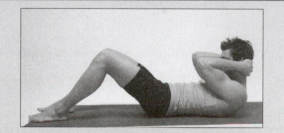

*d*o not elevate the upper body higher than the base of the shoulders in exercises such as Ab Curls, Half Roll-up, or Single Leg Stretch. The shoulder blades should be barely off the mat. In the photograph above the student has lifted his head and shoulders too high from the mat.

In the photograph above right the student is pulling on his neck and not allowing the elbows to remain open. To avoid pulling on the back of the neck when lifting the head for abdominal work, place the fingertips lightly on the base of the skull and do not intertwine them at the back of the head. Avoid poking or tucking the chin when lifting the head.

In the photograph at right the student has lost

his neutral spine position in the Connecting Navel to Spine fundamental exercise. His back is too arched and his head is out of alignment. It is important to be able to maintain a precise contraction of the inner core, keeping optimal form and spinal posture, before adding movements of the legs and arms.

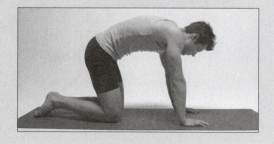

31

Half Roll-up with Arm Stretch and Tabletop Legs

After you have mastered the Ab Curls with Small Ball, make the exercise more interesting and progressively harder by adding an arm stretch and a lift of both legs. First, if you have no neck tension take the hands away from the back of the neck. Stretching the arms back from the body, slightly in front of the ears, adds a lever and challenges the abdominals. Lifting the legs to a tabletop position, with the knees and hips flexed at 90 degrees, increases the workload. Note that when the legs come up in the air in movement 3 the low back moves out of neutral and presses down gently on the mat. Remember to send the breath into the back of the rib cage.

Purpose To strengthen the abdominals and flatten the abdomen.

Watchpoints • Make sure you are strong enough to perform movement 3. • When the arms stretch back take extra care to make sure the shoulders are sliding downward, not up toward the ears. • When the arms are overhead keep an awareness of the link between rib cage and abdominals; do not let your back arch and your ribs pop out. • If the tabletop leg position creates too much work on the abdominals bring the knees in closer to the chest.

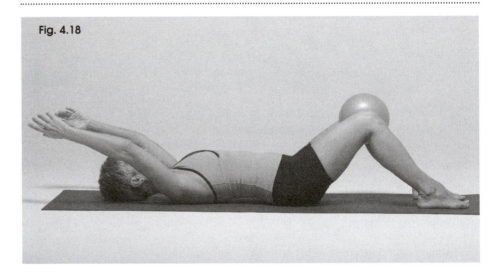

Fig. 4.18

starting position
Lie on your back, pelvis in neutral. Place the small ball between your knees. Start with the arms stretched slightly overhead (fig. 4.18).

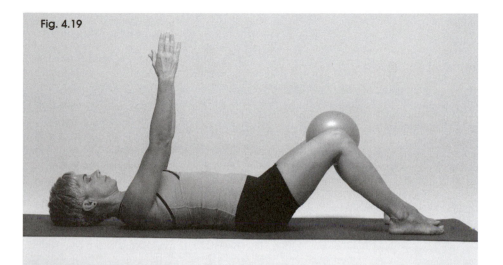

Fig. 4.19

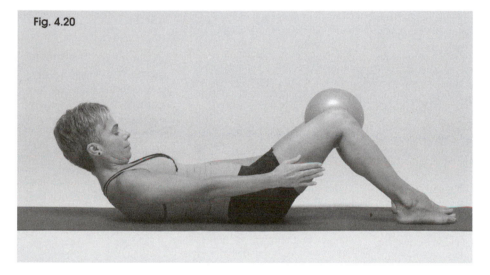

Fig. 4.20

movement 1: without arm stretch

1. Inhale to raise the hands toward the ceiling, keeping the shoulders down (fig. 4.19).

2. Exhale to sink the navel toward the spine and curl the upper body, bring-ing your hands to your thighs. Keep the pelvis in neutral (fig. 4.20).

3. Inhale and stay.

4. Exhale to roll back to the mat; arms return overhead.

5. Repeat six to eight times.

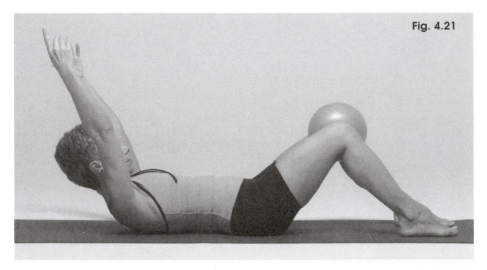

Fig. 4.21

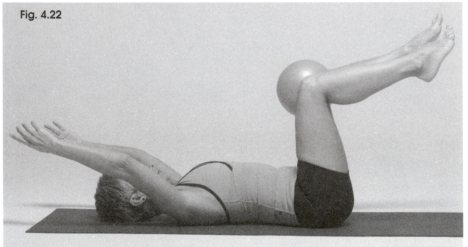

Fig. 4.22

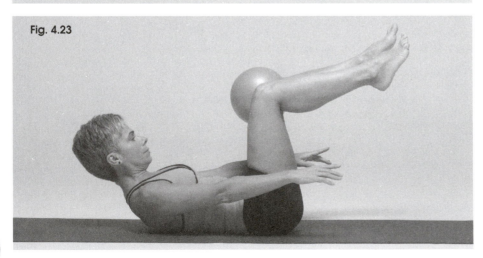

Fig. 4.23

movement 2: with arm stretch

1. Inhale to raise the arms toward the ceiling.

2. Exhale to sink the navel toward the spine and curl up, bringing the hands to your thighs. Your gaze is on your knees.

3. Inhaling, move the arms back slightly in front of the ears, keeping the body curled (fig. 4.21).

4. Exhale to roll back to the mat; arms return overhead.

5. Repeat six to eight times.

movement 3: add tabletop legs

1. Start with arms stretched overhead. Lift legs to table-top position (fig. 4.22).

2. Inhale to raise the arms toward the ceiling.

3. Exhale to sink the navel toward the spine and curl up, bringing the hands to your thighs. Make sure that your low back flattens to the mat (fig. 4.23).

4. Inhale and stay. Your gaze is on your knees, not the ceiling.

5. Exhale to roll back to the mat, arms overhead. If possible keep legs in tabletop position.

6. Repeat six to eight times.

Small Extensions on Small Ball

It is important to balance the curling forward of the spine with movements that open up the body. For this exercise use a very soft small ball with half the air let out of it, or use no ball at all. An extremely soggy ball will support the hips, relieve a sensitive low back, and help you feel whether your pelvis is steady. If the deep, stabilizing muscles are not working your pelvis will wobble from side to side. In movements 3 and 4 pull in your navel on the exhalation and engage the pelvic floor muscles as you add small, precise movements of the legs and arms. Make sure that the ball is positioned under the pelvis (across the hip-bones), not under the navel and upper abdomen. To understand how deflated the small ball should be for this exercise, compare the extremely soggy ball in figure 4.28 (page 37) to the fully inflated ball beside it.

Purpose To practice connecting navel to spine. To extend the spine and tone the buttocks and back of the legs.

Watchpoints • Make sure the pelvis does not move and that the buttocks remain relaxed in movements 1 and 2. • In the Single Leg Extension the buttocks will work as you stretch one leg two inches from the mat. Try to keep the opposite hipbone down to anchor the pelvis. • Keep the shoulders down and the neck long. Inhale into the back ribs; exhale to engage deep core muscles.

Modification • If you have knee problems avoid movement 5, the Shell Stretch. Curl up on your side instead.

starting position

Lie on your belly with a small ball with half the air let out of it nestled under your pelvis. Place one hand on top of the other and rest the forehead on the hands. Legs are extended on the mat and slightly turned out hip-distance apart. Toes are long.

movement 1: connecting navel to spine

1. Inhale to lengthen your body along the mat. Forehead remains on the mat (fig. 4.24).
2. Exhale to lift the navel. Remember this is a minuscule movement.
3. Inhale to release the navel.
4. Repeat six times.

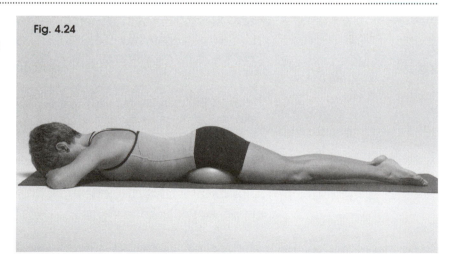

Fig. 4.24

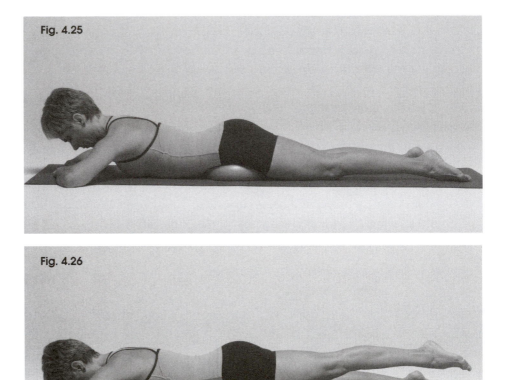

Fig. 4.25

Fig. 4.26

movement 2: small extension

1. Inhale to lengthen your body along the mat. Forehead is resting on the hands.
2. Exhale to lift navel and elongate and lift the upper body. Keep hands on the mat. Your gaze is on the mat (fig. 4.25).
3. Inhale and stay. Exhale to elongate your body back to the mat.
4. Repeat six times.

movement 3: single leg extensions

1. Keeping your head on the mat, inhale to stretch the left foot along the mat.
2. Exhale to lift the navel and extend the left foot two inches above the mat. Keep the leg very straight; you should

feel both buttocks at work (fig. 4.26).
3. Inhale to lower the left foot to the mat. Keep the abdominals connected. Try to keep the navel lifted; try not to let tension out of the muscle.
4. Exhale to lift the right foot two inches. Keep the leg straight and the pelvis steady.
5. Inhale to lower the right foot to the floor.
6. Repeat six times for each leg.

movement 4: single arm extensions

1. Inhale to glide the shoulder blades down as you extend the right arm along the mat. The other hand remains at your forehead.

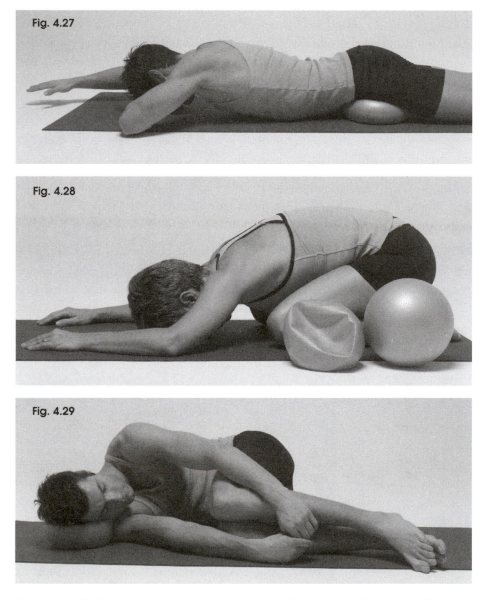

Fig. 4.27

Fig. 4.28

Fig. 4.29

2. Exhale to lift the right arm a couple of inches. Make sure the navel is pulled up. Head remains on the arm (fig. 4.27).
3. Inhale and stay.
4. Exhale to return the hand to the mat.
5. Repeat on the same side five times and then change arms.

movement 5: shell stretch

1. To stretch out the back, push against the mat with your hands to lift the body and sink back so that the back of the thighs come close to the buttocks (fig. 4.28).
2. If you have knee problems, curl up on the side of your body in a fetal position, a position known as Side Shell (fig. 4.29). Rest the side of your head on your arm or on the soggy ball.
3. Inhale through your nose to expand the back of the rib cage.
4. Exhale through your mouth to release.
5. Take five breaths, slow and deep.

Half Roll Down

The Half Roll Down teaches you to gently drop your navel into your spine and to control rolling through the spine with your abdominals. The small ball placed at the low back gives you sensory feedback. As you drop your navel into your spine to activate the abdominals, the low back presses against the ball. Imagine you're sinking your navel directly into the soft ball. Then a small rotation is added to challenge the oblique muscles. If you keep both exercises smooth, the small ball should remain in place at the base of your spine.

Purpose To strengthen abdominals and learn to keep these muscles flat. Movement 2 targets the obliques. To practice connecting navel to spine and prepare for rolling through the spine.

Watchpoints • Lead with the low back, not the upper back. • Keep shoulder blades sliding down. • Watch that your abdominals are connected and not bulging out, especially when you rotate to the front after the oblique twist.

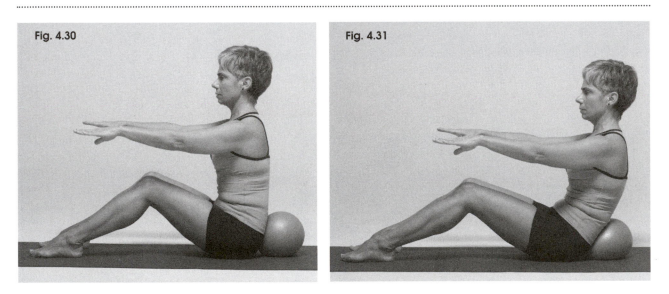

Fig. 4.30

Fig. 4.31

starting position

Sit tall on the mat with your legs parallel and hip-distance apart. Feet are planted firmly on the mat and not too close to the buttocks. Place the small ball at the base of your spine.

movement 1: half roll down

1. Inhale to lengthen through the spine, feeling as tall as possible (fig. 4.30).

2. Exhale to sink in your navel and roll off your sitz bones, curling the pelvis and letting the low back sink into the ball (fig. 4.31).
3. Inhale and stay.
4. Exhale to sink the navel deeper, keeping the upper body where it is.
5. Inhale to return to a tall sitting position.
6. Repeat six to eight times.

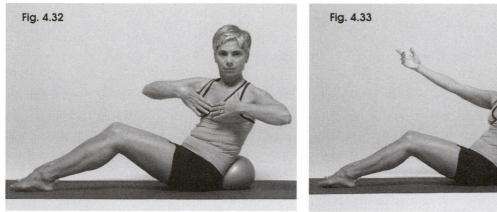

Fig. 4.32 Fig. 4.33

movement 2: half roll down with obliques

1. Inhale to lengthen through the spine, feeling as tall as possible. Hands are at your heart, elbows open and lifted.

2. Exhale to sink in your navel and roll off your sitz bones, curling your pelvis and leading with the low back.

3. Keeping your body where it is, inhale to rotate, hands at the heart (fig. 4.32).

4. Exhale to maintain the C-curve by keeping the navel pulled in as you open the arms (fig. 4.33).

5. Inhaling, place your hands back at the heart, elbows lifted.

6. Exhale to rotate back to center. Check that the navel is pulled in.

7. Inhale to return to tall sitting position.

8. Repeat six to eight times, rotating from side to side.

Whole-body Movement

*a*n exercise system that worked only the abdominals would be an unhealthy regime. A ball can be used to train a muscle in isolation; however, more often than not pitting your gravity-bound body against a mobile ball forces the entire body to work. This is why the ball is so useful in rehabilitating motor learning as well as enhancing ordinary or elite fitness. Unlike traditional mat or machine exercises, working on a ball develops what physiotherapists call "coordinative structures," because one body part is not being trained in isolation of another.

Exercise machines support the back and buttocks, which often means that these areas relax during a workout and are not recruited for performing the exercise. On the ball, muscles keep working. Physical therapist and exercise ball pioneer Joanne Posner-Mayer uses exercises to help her patients acquire new and more flexible motor skills. She explains how standing on one foot while "trapping" a ball with the other foot as one writes the letters of the alphabet with the toes on the surface of the ball utilizes deep and superficial muscles necessary for keeping the body upright. This exercise challenges proprioception (the sensory feedback mechanism that tells the body where it is in space) and imitates the same motor activity required to avoid a fall. Working the body in its entirety is essential for achieving healthy functional movement.

Rolling Like a Ball

This time you will roll down and up, massaging the spine and controlling the movement with the abdominals. Using the small ball to focus the movement and keep the legs connected, start by rolling just to the back of the sitz bones. If possible keep the feet off the mat the whole time, creating a challenge for balance and for the abdominals. Later, if desired, try the large ball on the shins. The large ball helps you keep your heels close to your buttocks to maintain the correct tight "ball" position, but it is considerably more difficult. Reverse the breath and find out what works best for you.

Purpose To control rolling through the spine with your abdominals.

Watchpoints • Keep your eyes focused on your knees so that the head does not touch the mat in the full movement. • Keep the shoulders sliding down the back; rest the hands in a relaxed manner on the legs. • Keep the heels close to the body. Sink the navel toward the spine to lead with the low back.

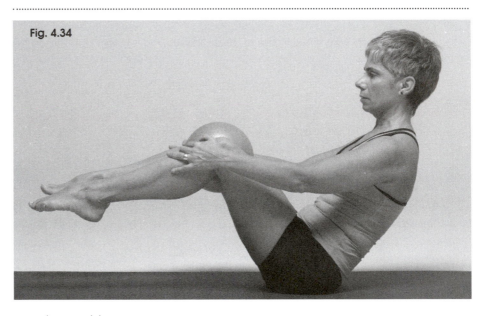

Fig. 4.34

starting position

Balance in a C-curve, leaning just to the back of your sitz bones. Place the small ball between your knees.

movement 1: without rolling back

1. Inhale to prepare. Feet are a couple of inches off the mat.
2. Exhale to drop the navel toward the

spine, keeping the body in a C-curve (fig. 4.34).
3. Inhale to return to starting position, keeping your curve shape.
4. Exhale to drop the navel—your abdominals keep you from rolling back. Feet should remain off the mat the entire time to increase difficulty and challenge.
5. Repeat five times.

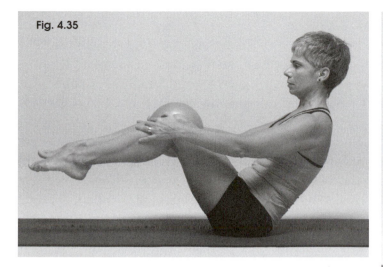

Fig. 4.35

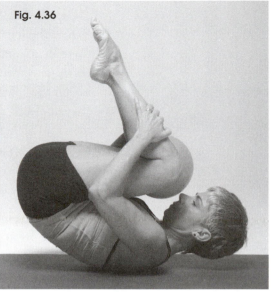

Fig. 4.36

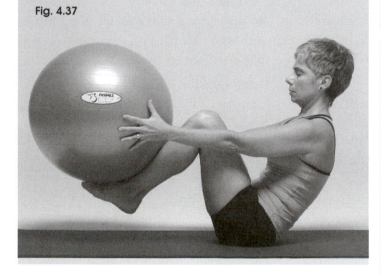

Fig. 4.37

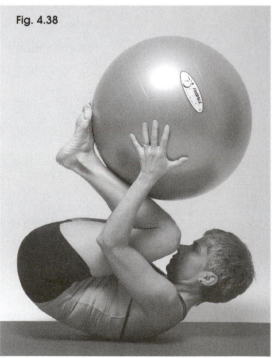

Fig. 4.38

movement 2: rolling like a ball

1. Start just at the back of the sitz bones, feet a couple of inches off the mat (fig. 4.35). Inhale.

2. Exhale to drop the navel toward the spine and roll back, leading with the low back (fig. 4.36).

3. Inhale to return to the starting position.

4. Exhale to roll back. Keep your gaze on the knees so the head does not fly back.

5. Repeat six to eight times.

movement 3: with large ball

1. Rest the large ball on your shins (fig. 4.37).

2. Reversing the breath, inhale to drop the navel toward the spine and roll back (fig. 4.38).

3. Exhale to return forward.

4. Repeat six to eight times.

Single Leg Stretch

When the legs are in the air, as they are in Single Leg Stretch, take care that the pelvis is stabilized and the low back is not arching excessively. When correctly executed the pelvis will move out of neutral and into a position in which the low back flattens, or gently imprints, onto the mat. In movement 4 the small ball rests between the shoulder blades to add support. Use the ball as a tool to help you experience the breath as it widens the back of the rib cage. As soon as you have mastered the coordination for this exercise we add a small squeeze to the ball during the exhale for upper-body resistance. Try squeezing the ball close to you as well as above your head. Finally, try passing the ball under the upper leg each time you extend the bottom leg.

Purpose To work on coordination, breathing, and abdominal strength.

Watchpoints • Keep ankles, knees, and hips in alignment. • Keep legs fully stretched, toes softly pointed. • The upper torso is stable; do not pull the shoulders from side to side or allow them to hunch up to your ears as you squeeze the ball. • Your gaze is on the knees, not on the ceiling.

Modification • If you have low-back pain keep the legs higher than 45 degrees as you extend them. If you have neck tension leave the head down on the mat.

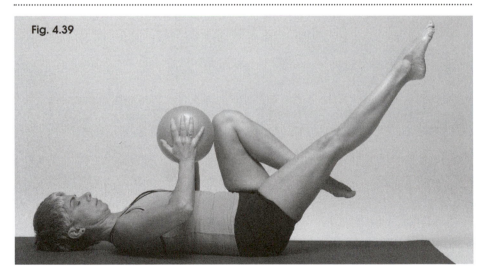

Fig. 4.39

starting position

Lie flat on your back, knees to chest. Hold the small ball on your knees.

movement 1: head down

1. Inhale to prepare, holding the small ball quite close to your chest. Elbows are bent.
2. Exhale to extend one leg, squeezing the ball (fig. 4.39).

3. Inhale to bring the legs back to the tabletop position.

4. Exhale to extend the second leg, squeezing the ball.

5. Repeat for five sets, or ten times with each leg.

movement 2: lifting the head

1. Inhale to prepare, holding the small ball on your knees (fig. 4.40).

2. Exhale to curl the upper body (fig. 4.41). as you simultaneously extend one leg 45 degrees from the floor. Place the small ball directly above your chest and squeeze. Gaze is on your knees, not on the ceiling (fig. 4.42).

3. Inhale to bring the legs back to tabletop position.

4. Exhale to stretch the other leg 45 degrees from the floor. Squeeze the small ball. Elbows are soft, not locked.

5. Inhale to switch, and exhale to extend the leg.

6. Repeat for five sets, or ten times with each leg.

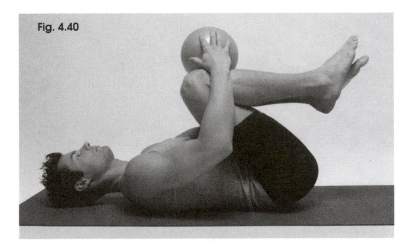

Fig. 4.40

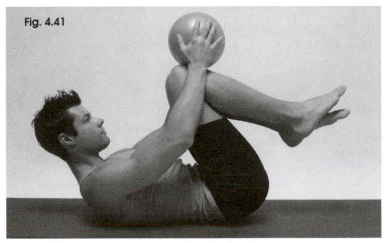

Fig. 4.41

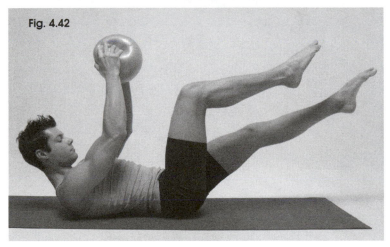

Fig. 4.42

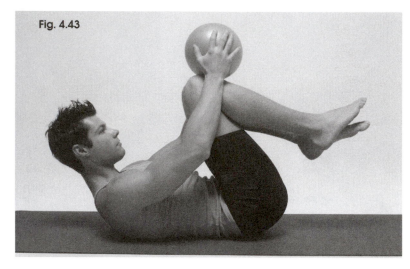

Fig. 4.43

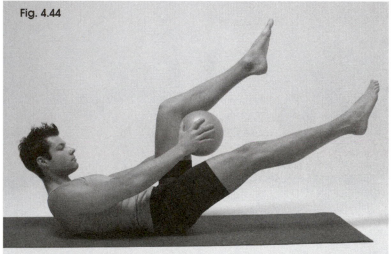

Fig. 4.44

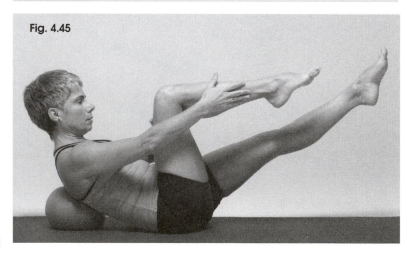

Fig. 4.45

movement 3: passing the ball under the leg

1. Inhale to prepare, holding the small ball on your knees.

2. Exhale to curl the upper body (fig. 4.43) as you simultaneously extend one leg 45 degrees from the floor. Pass the ball under the top bent leg (fig. 4.44). Gaze is on your knees, not on the ceiling.

3. Inhale to bring the legs back to table-top position.

4. Exhale to stretch the other leg 45 degrees from the floor. Pass the ball under the top bent leg.

5. Inhale to switch, and exhale to extend the leg.

6. Repeat for five sets, or ten times with each leg.

movement 4: with small ball support

1. Place the small ball between or just under the shoulder blades. Curl the upper body and lift the knees, placing your hands on your knees. Don't sink the low back into the ball; rather, lift your body slightly off the ball. You should feel your abdominals engage in this position. Inhale.

2. Exhale to extend your left leg. Bring your right hand to the ankle and your left hand to the knee of the bent leg (fig. 4.45).

3. Inhale to bring the legs back to table-top position.

4. Exhale to extend your right leg. Bring the left hand to the ankle and the right hand to the knee of the bent leg.

5. Repeat for five sets, or ten times with each leg.

Oblique Twists

This can be done with a soggy 55-cm ball or a small ball. Do not neglect these and the other oblique exercises. Well-toned obliques present a slim waist and enhance the performance of many sports that use twisting movements. Gently squeezing the ball between the knees targets the inner thighs and the muscles deep in the pelvic floor. Take care when you squeeze not to allow the tail to curl up. Try to perform this exercise slowly and precisely, keeping the pelvis in neutral. With each exhalation think of sliding the rib cage toward the opposite hipbone. Keep the elbows reaching out to the sides.

Purpose To tone the oblique muscles and the inner thighs.

Watchpoints • Hands are placed lightly behind the ears; elbows reach to the side. • Keep the tailbone on the mat and try not to rock the pelvis. • Keep the abdominals flat and hollowed.

starting position

Lie on your back with the ball positioned between your knees. Feet remain flat on the mat. Hands are behind the ears, elbows wide. Hands can be on the forehead (fig. 4.46).

movement 1: oblique twist

1. Inhale to prepare.
2. Keeping your pelvis in neutral, exhale as you pin your right elbow back and bring your left rib cage across the body, all the while gently squeezing the ball (fig. 4.47).
3. Inhale to lie the head back on the mat.
4. Exhale to pin the left elbow and bring the right side of the rib cage across the body as you gently squeeze the ball.
5. Repeat eight to ten times on each side.

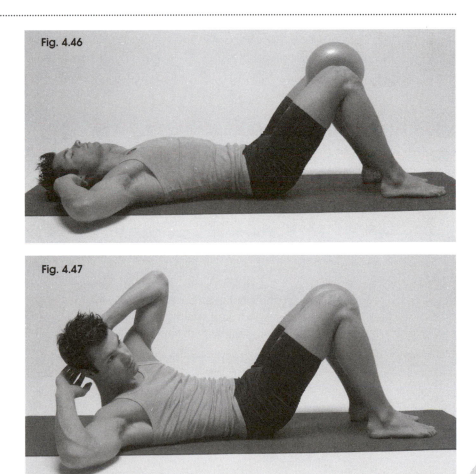

Fig. 4.46

Fig. 4.47

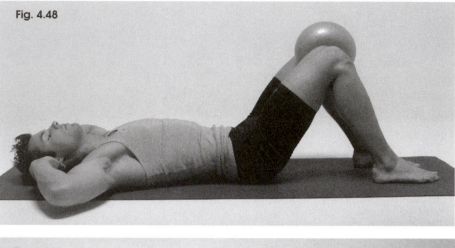

Fig. 4.48

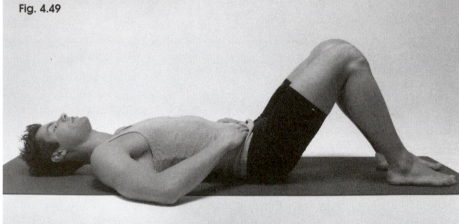

Fig. 4.49

movement 2: just squeeze

1. Keep your head on the mat. Inhale to release the ball.
2. Exhale to squeeze the ball, isolating the inner thigh but not allowing the tailbone to curl upward (fig. 4.48).
3. Repeat eight times.

movement 3: check in with the deep abdominals

1. From the same starting position, place your three longest fingers one inch in from the hipbones on the front of the pelvis and press. Keep the pelvis in neutral.
2. Inhale to release the ball.
3. Exhale to squeeze the ball gently, isolating the inner thigh but not allowing the tailbone to curl upward (fig. 4.49). Can you feel tension on your fingertips as the deep transversus abdominis is activated?
4. Repeat eight times.

Sidework with Small Ball

Now we roll onto the side and position the body so that the neck, shoulders, hips, and knees are in the same line. Hips will be stacked one on top of the other, and it will be the navel-to-spine connection that stabilizes the hips. If possible try not to sink through the rib cage; keep the waist off the mat. Tighten the pelvic floor and think of initiating the movement from the abdominals.

Purpose To work the abdominals, inner and outer thighs, and gluteals.

Watchpoints • Do not look down at your feet; look straight out in front of you. • Do not lift the legs too high; you should not feel pain in your waist. • Check to see that the kneecaps and hips are facing forward. • Do not sink the waist into the mat. Keep the abs flat and the upper body relaxed.

starting position

Lie on your side in a long line from the head through the shoulders, hips, and feet. Your head can be propped up by your hand or relaxed on the mat. Square your shoulders and use the hand in front for support. Lift your upper body up and out of the waist.

movement 1: thigh squeeze

1. Place a soggy small ball between your thighs. Inhale to prepare.
2. Exhale to squeeze the ball (fig. 4.50).
3. Repeat eight times. Keep the body long and stable.

movement 2: press top leg

1. Place a small ball between the ankles. Inhale to prepare.
2. Exhale to press the top leg down on the small ball (fig. 4.51).
3. Repeat eight times. Keep the body long and stable.

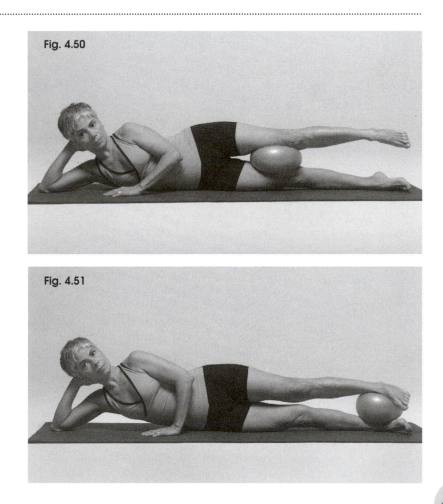

Fig. 4.50

Fig. 4.51

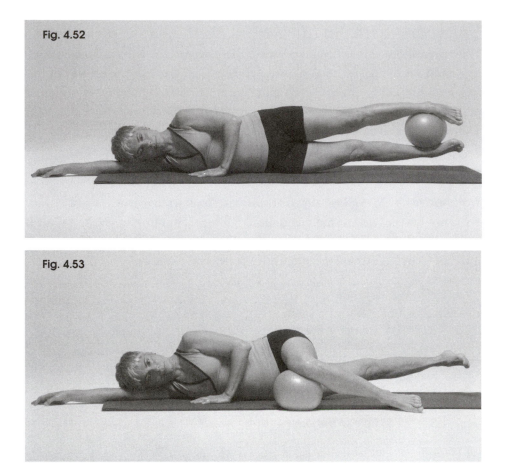

Fig. 4.52

Fig. 4.53

movement 3: ankle squeeze and lift

1. Keep the small ball between the ankles. Release your upper body to the mat, extending your right arm and resting your head on your arm.
2. Inhale to prepare.
3. Exhale to squeeze both legs together and lift both legs a couple of inches (fig. 4.52).
4. Inhale to lower. Exhale to lift.
5. Repeat eight times. Keep the body long and stable.

movement 4: inner thigh circles

1. To isolate the inner thigh of the bottom leg, bring the top leg across mid-line. Prop the ball under the top knee to ensure alignment of the pelvis, then completely relax the top leg and focus on the inner thigh of the bottom leg.
2. Inhale to flex the bottom foot and straighten the heel away from you. Pulse the leg up and down. Keep the leg very straight and exhale on the lift for ten pulses (fig. 4.53).
3. Then, keeping the abdominals and pelvic floor contracted, lift the leg a couple of inches. Leading with the heel, make six rapid small circles in one direction and six in the other direction.
4. Repeat the entire Sidework series on the other side.

Hip Rolls with Small Ball

Squeezing the small ball between the knees is an excellent way to feel the engagement of the pelvic floor and the abdominals. The hamstrings (the muscles on the back of the legs) and the gluteals will also be at work. A gentle squeeze on the ball is all that is necessary. Raising the arms overhead takes away from your base of support, adding to the challenge. This is a sequencing exercise; try to imagine the vertebrae moving individually, not in a chunk.

Purpose To strengthen abdominals, buttocks, and back of the legs. To teach core stability.

Watchpoints • Do not overarch at the top of the exercise. • In the top position maintain a straight line through your knees, hips, and shoulders. Your weight is equally supported on both feet.

....

starting position

Lie on your back with your knees bent and your feet flat on the floor, hip-distance apart. The pelvis is in neutral. Place the small ball between your knees. Rest your hands by your sides; shoulders are sliding down away from the ears.

movement 1: ordinary hip roll

1. Inhale to lengthen the tailbone away from the pelvis.
2. Exhale to drop the navel and lengthen the low back on the mat, then curl the pelvis upward. Your buttocks should squeeze together gently. The pelvic floor is engaged (fig. 4.54).
3. Inhale at the top.
4. Exhale to soften through the chest and sequence down one vertebra at a time, pressing the low back on the mat and coming back to neutral pelvis.
5. Repeat four times.

movement 2: with arm stretch

1. Inhale to lengthen the tailbone away from the pelvis.
2. Exhale to drop the navel and lengthen the low back on the mat, then curl the pelvis upward. Your buttocks should squeeze together gently. The pelvic floor is engaged.
3. Inhale at the top, lifting the arms and taking them overhead (fig. 4.55).

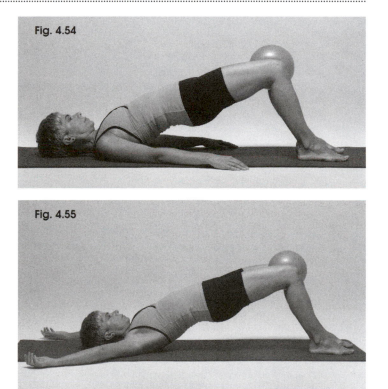

Fig. 4.54

Fig. 4.55

4. Leave the arms overhead as you exhale to soften through the chest and sequence down one vertebra at a time, pressing the low back on the mat and coming back to neutral pelvis.
5. Repeat four times.

Hips Rolls with Leg Extensions

These hip rolls are in the same family as the previous exercise but are much more challenging. Holding the hips up in the air for ten seconds or longer while maintaining the abdominal contraction is an excellent way to train the deep core. Do not forget to breathe while you hold up the hips. Make sure the abdominals and gluteals are working to support the heavy pelvis so you do not feel discomfort in the low back. For movement 2, maintain a straight line through the knees, hips, and shoulders as you take one leg off the mat and extend it.

Purpose To strengthen the abdominals, buttocks, and back of legs. To teach core stability.

Watchpoints • Do not overarch at the top. • Keep the pelvis steady; do not allow the hip to drop or twist when you extend the leg. • Keep the upper body relaxed.

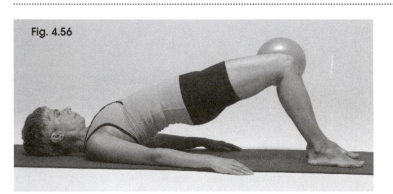

Fig. 4.56

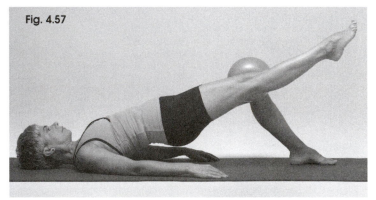

Fig. 4.57

starting position

Lie on your back with your knees bent and your feet flat on the floor, hip-distance apart. The pelvis is in neutral.

Place the small ball between your knees. Rest your hands by your side; shoulders are sliding down away from the ears.

movement 1: hold contraction

1. Inhale to lengthen the tailbone away from the pelvis.
2. Exhale to drop the navel and lengthen the low back on the mat, then curl the pelvis upward. Your buttocks should squeeze together gently. The pelvic floor is engaged.
3. Remain with the pelvis in the air for ten seconds, breathing naturally (fig. 4.56).
4. Repeat four times, holding for 10 to 15 seconds. Do not hold your breath.

movement 2: with leg extension

1. Inhale to lengthen the tailbone away from the pelvis.
2. Exhale to drop the navel and lengthen the low back on the mat, then curl the pelvis upward. Your buttocks should squeeze together gently. The pelvic floor is engaged.
3. Inhale at the top.
4. Keeping the pelvis steady and the small ball in place, exhale to extend one leg (fig. 4.57).
5. Inhale to place the foot back on the mat.
6. Exhale to extend the other leg.
7. Inhale to return the leg to the mat.
8. Exhale to soften through the chest and sequence down one vertebra at a time, pressing the low back on the mat and coming back to neutral pelvis.
9. Repeat four times on each leg.

Ab Curls on Small Ball

Diversity is important when training the abdominals. The shape of the ball allows for a greater range of movement than a mat, and the small ball acts as a support for beginners who may not be steady enough to perform these exercises on a large ball. Here is a chance for the abdominals to lengthen out instead of just crunching forward. Do not flex too high. Sink the navel toward the spine and keep the pelvis in neutral as you hold the contraction and then work the obliques.

Purpose To strengthen upper abdominals. Movement 3 challenges the obliques.

Watchpoints • Keep your pelvis stable and in neutral. • Do not sink the waist and take care that the back does not arch. • Do not pull on your neck or jam your chin into your chest.

starting position

Lie on the mat and place the small ball between your shoulder blades or slightly below the blades. Bend your knees; place the feet in line with the knees and the knees in line with the hips. Buttocks remain on the mat. Place your hands lightly behind your ears to support your head (fig. 4.58).

movement 1: curls

1. Inhale to prepare, keeping the elbows reaching to the sides.
2. Exhale to pull in your navel and curl the upper body. The tops of the shoulder blades will come off the ball (fig. 4.59).
3. Inhale and stay.

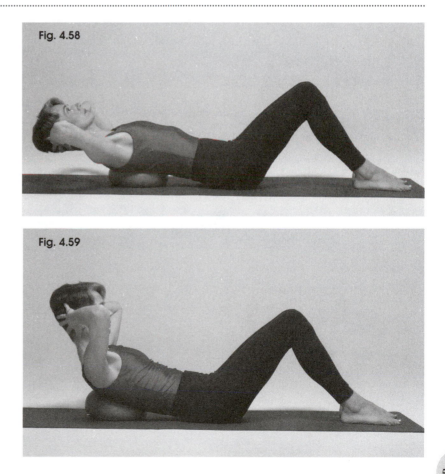

Fig. 4.58

Fig. 4.59

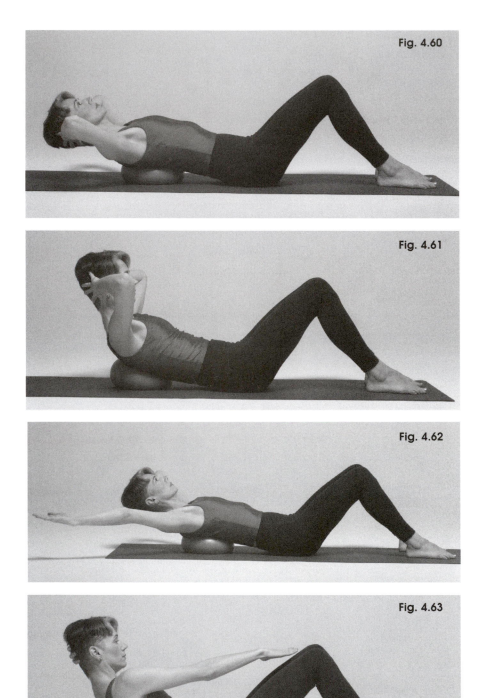

Fig. 4.60

Fig. 4.61

Fig. 4.62

Fig. 4.63

4. Exhale to lower, lengthening your upper body over the ball (fig. 4.60). Feel the abdominals stretch.

5. Repeat eight times, slow and controlled.

movement 2: hold contraction

1. Inhale to prepare, keeping the elbows reaching to the sides.

2. Exhale to pull in your navel and curl the upper body. The tops of the shoulder blades will come off the ball.

3. Inhale, exhale, and inhale slowly to hold the contraction for 3 to 4 seconds (fig. 4.61).

4. Exhale to lower, lengthening your upper body over the ball. Feel the abdominals stretch.

5. Repeat six times, slow and controlled.

movement 3: add oblique twist

1. Place one hand behind the head and stretch the other hand overhead. Inhale to pre-pare (fig. 4.62).

2. Exhale to pull in the navel and curl the body, bringing the working hand to the opposite knee (fig. 4.63). The other hand continues to support the head.

3. Inhale to lower, lengthening your upper body over the ball. Feel the abdominals stretch.

4. Repeat eight times on the same side, slow and controlled.

5. Change sides to repeat the exercise.

The Waterfall

The abdominals and the hip flexors work when rolling the ball, small or large, up and over the knees to the ankles. Just go as far as you are able, and avoid this exercise if you have low-back pain. Keep your shoulders stabilized when you roll the ball along the trunk and the legs: don't let the position of the hands on the ball cause the shoulders to lift toward the ears. Watch that your elbows stay slightly bent as you push the ball up the thighs. Try not to just "go through the motions"—notice how the pelvis moves out of neutral and the low back pushes gently downward on the mat as you roll up and roll down though the spine. The ball slows the movement and helps you focus on each bone as it makes contact with the mat.

Purpose To strengthen the abdominal muscles. The hip flexors will also be at work in this exercise.

Watchpoints • The ball stays in contact with the body. • Keep the abdomen flat and hollowed; remember to connect navel to spine, and do not arch the low back when you roll up or down. • Keep the shoulders down and back.

Modification • Avoid this exercise if you experience pain in the low back. Keep the knees bent and do a Half Roll-up instead.

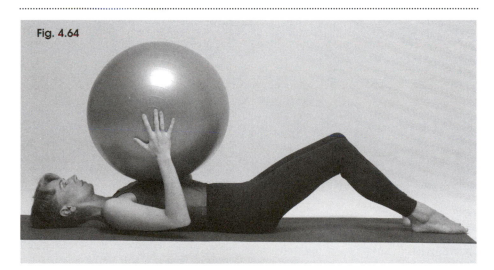

Fig. 4.64

starting position

Lie on your back with knees bent and feet on the floor, hip-distance apart.
Place the ball on the rib cage with one hand on each side of the ball. Be sure that the feet are not too close to the buttocks (fig. 4.64).

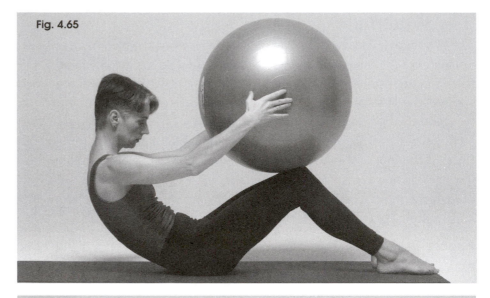

Fig. 4.65

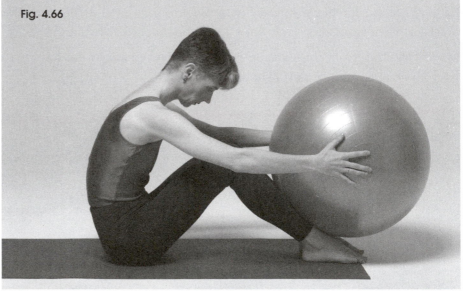

Fig. 4.66

movement: the waterfall

1. Inhale to lengthen on the mat.
2. Exhale to lift the head and flex the upper body as you roll the ball up the thighs (fig. 4.65). over the knees, and down the shins. Release the head (fig. 4.66).

3. Inhale when the ball is at the ankles as you begin to roll back.
4. Exhale to sink the navel and reverse the movement, rolling down one vertebra at a time, eventually releasing the head to the mat.
5. Repeat six to eight times, slow and controlled.

Hip Rolls on Large Ball

You will now change the body's relationship with gravity by placing the legs on the large ball. Take care with both Hip Roll exercises that, when you return the pelvis to the mat, you do not exaggerate the curve in the low back by forcing down the tailbone and making a larger space in the low back than is beneficial. The farther the ball is from the torso the more difficult the exercise.

Purpose To sequence through the body and create mobility in the spine. To strengthen buttock muscles and the core.

Watchpoints • Do not overarch at the top: lift the pelvis only a couple of inches if you have moderate low-back pain. • Connect through the inner thighs; try not to let the legs separate on the ball. • The neck and shoulders should be relaxed.

starting position

Lie on your back with your calf muscles resting on the ball and your hands on either side of your thighs. Connect through the inner thighs. Be sure that the shoulders are sliding down away from your ears (fig. 4.67).

movement 1: ordinary hip roll

1. Inhale to lengthen the tailbone away from the pelvis.
2. Exhale to drop the navel and imprint the low back on the mat, then curve the tailbone and lift the pelvis until your body is in a straight line, shoulders in line with toes (fig. 4.68).
3. Inhale at the top.
4. Exhale to soften through the chest and sequence down one vertebra at a time.
5. Repeat four times.

movement 2: hold pelvis in air

1. Inhale to lengthen the tailbone away from the pelvis.
2. Exhale to drop the navel and imprint the low back on the mat, then curve the tailbone and lift the pelvis until your body is in a straight line, shoulders in line with toes.
3. Inhale at the top and continue to breathe naturally as you hold the pelvis steady in the air for 15 to 20 seconds (fig. 4.68).

4. Exhale to sequence the body back to the mat.
5. Repeat twice.

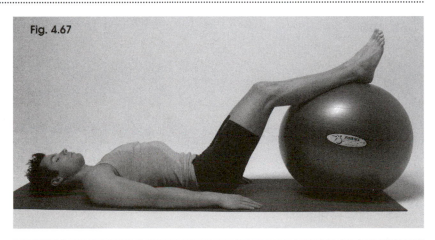
Fig. 4.67

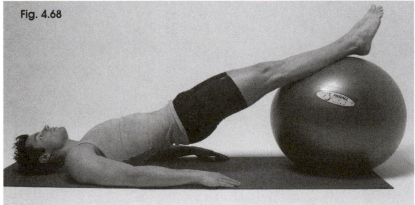
Fig. 4.68

Hip Rolls with Balance

Attempt this balance only when your body is feeling strong and pain free. Once you have mastered Hip Rolls, roll the ball to the ankles so that you can create a long, straight line from the shoulders through the hips and knees to your toes. Remember that the more challenging you make the exercise the harder it is to maintain the deep abdominal contraction. In this exercise we are testing the core strength of the body by decreasing the solid base of support. The stabilizers must be very strong or you may roll off the ball completely.

Purpose To strengthen the core and test balance.

Watchpoints • Do not overarch at the top by lifting the pelvis too high. • Be sure your neck is relaxed.

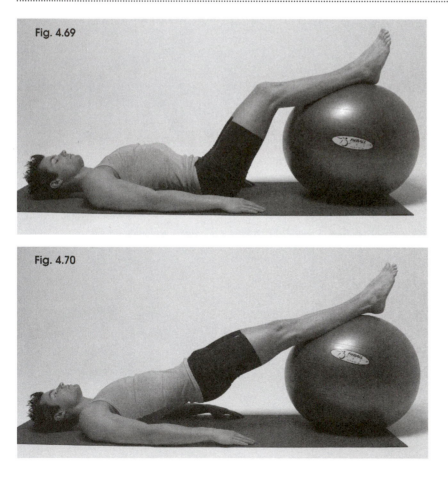

Fig. 4.69

Fig. 4.70

starting position

Lie on your back with your calves or ankles resting on the ball and hands on either side of your thighs. Connect through the inner thighs. Be sure that the shoulders are sliding down away from your ears (fig. 4.69).

movement 1: lift wrists

1. Inhale to lengthen the tailbone away from the pelvis.
2. Exhale to continue to lengthen and curl the tailbone one vertebra at a time until your body is in a straight line, shoulders in line with toes (fig. 4.70).
3. Hold this position, breathing normally and connecting through the buttocks, inner thighs, and abdominals.

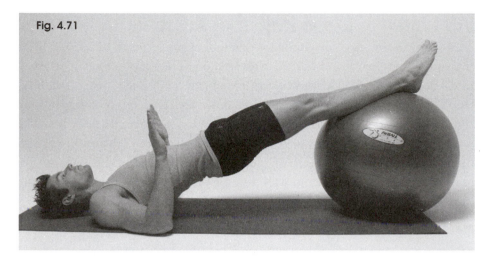

Fig. 4.71

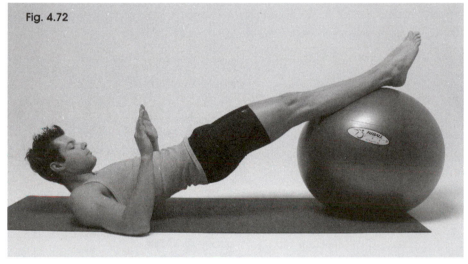

Fig. 4.72

4. Leaving elbows on the mat, slowly lift the wrists and hands off the mat. Breathe naturally and hold for a few counts (fig. 4.71).
5. Exhale to soften through the chest and sequence down one vertebra at a time.

movement 2: lift head

1. Follow instructions for movement 1, this time lifting the head off the mat for extra challenge. Breathe naturally and hold for a few counts (fig. 4.72).
2. Replace the head on the mat. Exhale to soften through the chest and sequence down one vertebra at a time.
3. Repeat this series twice.

Ab Curls on Large Ball

This is one of the most pleasurable abdominal exercises you'll ever do; it feels like doing exercises on a waterbed. Research published in the June 2000 issue of *Physical Therapy* concludes that abdominal curls performed on a mobile surface are much more effective than those done on a mat, as the instability of the ball increases the muscle activity and the way the muscles coactivate to stablize the spine and the whole body. Use the ball to your advantage by noting how the abdominals stretch and lengthen as you perform the exercise. To make the exercise less difficult, walk your feet a few steps in front of the ball, dropping the buttocks slightly.

Purpose To strengthen the upper and superficial abdominals.

Watchpoints • Make sure to keep your buttocks lifted to the same height as the thighs and knees. • Keep your torso stable. • Do not pull on your neck. • Do not push your chin into your chest when you curl up.

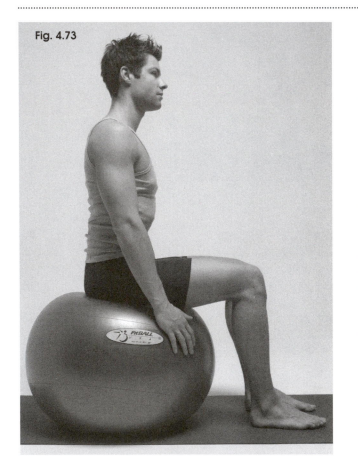

Fig. 4.73

starting position

Sit on the center of your ball (fig. 4.73). Slowly walk your feet away from the ball; the ball will roll under you. Walk the feet out until the shoulders are resting comfortably on the ball. Place the hands behind the ears (fig. 4.74).

movement 1: hips up

1. Inhale to prepare, keeping the elbows reaching to the side.
2. Exhale to pull your navel in and curl the upper body. The lower back is off the ball (fig. 4.75).
3. Inhale and stay.
4. Exhale to lower the upper body to the ball.
5. Inhale to lengthen back, feeling the abdominals stretch.
6. Repeat eight times, slow and controlled.

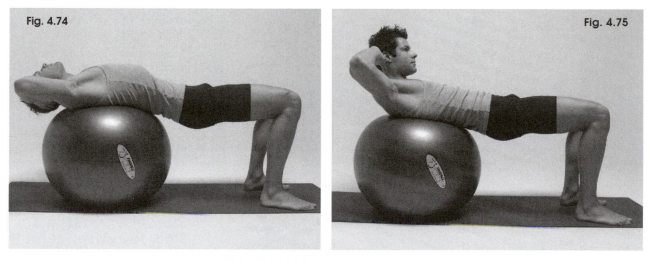

Fig. 4.74

Fig. 4.75

movement 2: oblique variation

1. Come into position in the same way as movement 1. The left arm is stretched out holding the small ball if desired. The other hand rests lightly on the base of the skull, behind the ear. Inhale to prepare (fig. 4.76).

2. Exhale to slide the rib cage toward the opposite hip as you extend the left arm across the body toward the right knee. Keep hips up (fig. 4.77).

3. Inhale to lie back on the ball.

4. Exhale to rotate across to the same side.

5. Repeat with eight repetitions on one side, then switch sides.

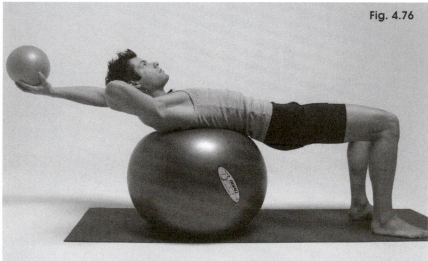

Fig. 4.76

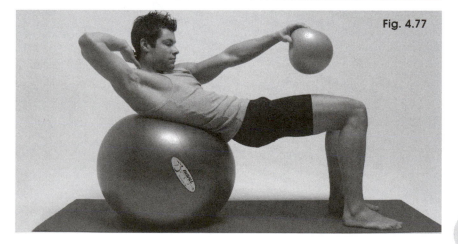

Fig. 4.77

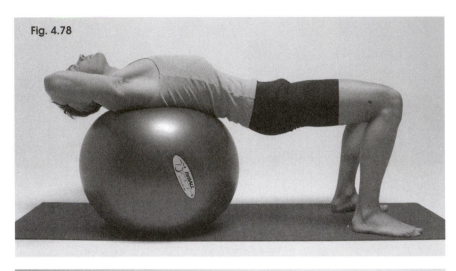

Fig. 4.78

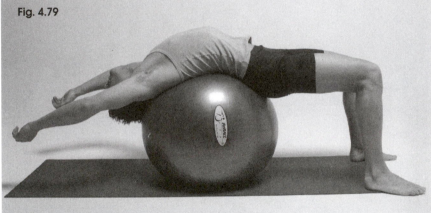

Fig. 4.79

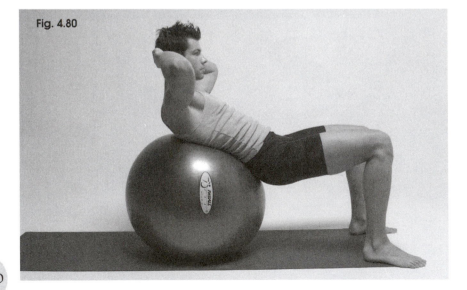

Fig. 4.80

movement 3: stretch out back and abdominals

1. Slowly walk your feet away from the ball, holding the head if desired (fig. 4.78). Continue to walk the feet until the head and neck are totally supported by the ball.

2. Gently lift the buttocks to keep the hips in line with the knees and shoulders. Open your arms to the side or overhead and stretch out the back and abdominals.

3. Stay here and breathe for a few counts (fig. 4.79).

4. To come out of the stretch, put your hands behind your head and immediately lift the head, chin to chest (fig. 4.80). Walk your feet slowly toward the ball as you begin to sit up. Place your hands on the top of the ball to aid you as you continue to walk your feet in and curl up until you are sitting back on the ball. This is not easy for beginners. You may have to lower your buttocks to the ground instead to come out of the exercise.

Walk Up and Down

Performing an abdominal curl while rolling on the ball will cause your abs to wake up and take notice. Moving the body from vertical to horizontal and back to vertical is not as easy as it looks in the photos—that is the reason the following exercise comes toward the end of the "Basic Abs on the Ball" chapter. Begin this exercise with your fingertips on the ball. Once you have the knack of this tricky move you can cross your hands over your chest or reach your arms straight out in front of you. Movement 3 adds the element of speed to the exercise. Joanne Posner-Mayer uses this exercise to mimic the body experience of losing and then recovering balance. She reminds us that this exercise is not just an abdominal isolator but also trains the muscles of the buttocks and the deep core muscles for supporting the spine.

Purpose To challenge the abdominals and core and to improve balance and coordination.

Watchpoints • Make sure you have enough traction to do this exercise: wear nonslip shoes if you feel yourself slipping. • Try not to let the buttocks drop and make sure the ball moves out in a straight line. • Protect the neck with the hands if you need to. • Keep feet flat on ground and resist the urge to go up on your toes.

starting position

Sit on the center of the ball. Feet are parallel, shoulder-distance apart. Start with fingertips on the ball (fig. 4.81).

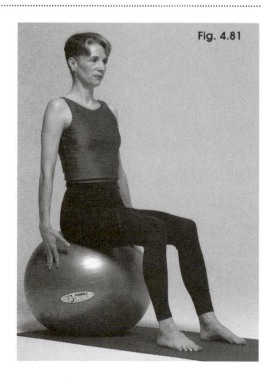

Fig. 4.81

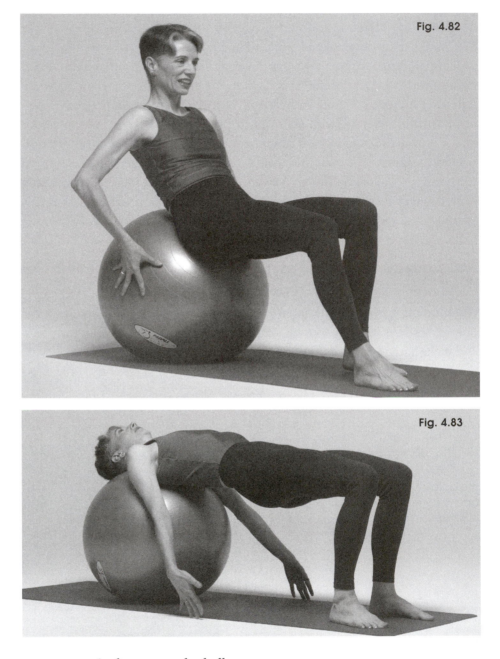

Fig. 4.82

Fig. 4.83

movement 1: fingers on the ball

1. Inhale as you slowly begin to walk your feet away from the ball.

2. Exhale to pull in the navel. As the ball rolls forward and you roll down your spine, continue to move your feet forward (fig. 4.82).

3. Keep walking, taking care to keep your buttocks up. The back will be straight. Walk out until your shoulders or neck rest on the ball. Squeeze the buttocks. The pelvis is lifted (fig. 4.83). You may need to support the neck with your hands. Inhale.

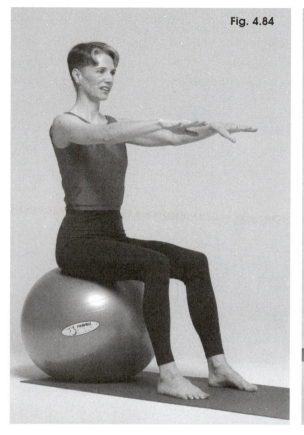

Fig. 4.84

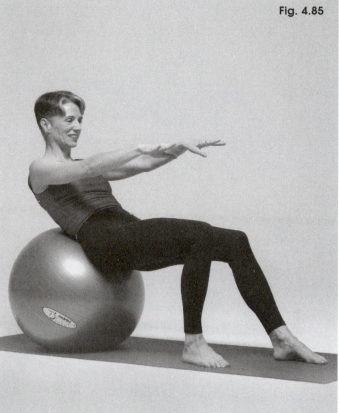

Fig. 4.85

4. Exhale to return, scooping the navel and walking slowly in reverse, curling your torso. Continue to walk until you are sitting tall on the ball. Keep fingers on the ball for assistance.
5. Repeat six times.

movement 2: hands off the ball

1. Hands are crossed over your chest or stretched in front of you (fig. 4.84). Perform the same movement as movement 1, but keep hands off the ball (fig. 4.85).
2. Repeat six times.

movement 3: add speed

1. When you are ready, perform the same movement as above but add the element of speed.
2. Repeat six times, moving as rapidly up and down as you can, keeping good technique and not letting the buttocks drop in the "lying down" phase of the exercise.

Rolling from Side to Side

This is a great exercise for challenging the obliques. Initiate the rotation from the core. Use the small ball to help focus the exercise and assist in stabilizing the shoulders. Feel the rotation in the spine—do not just extend through the arms. Keep the pelvis square to the front.

Purpose To challenge the obliques and to improve balance and coordination.

Watchpoints • Avoid sidebending. • Keep elbows and hands in one line. • Do not let the shoulders round forward; keep open across the collarbones.

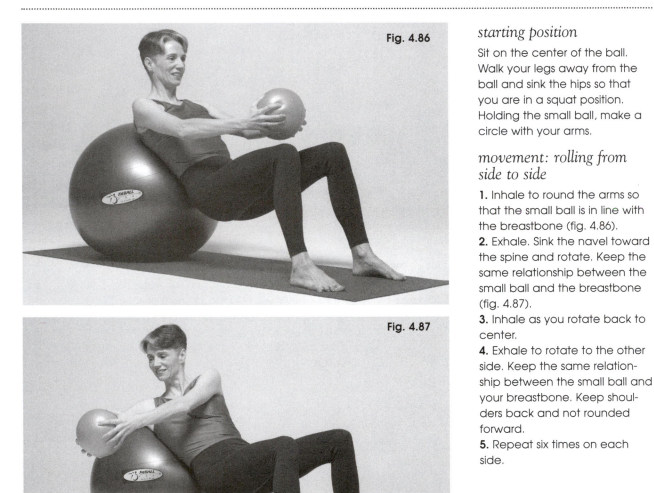

Fig. 4.86

Fig. 4.87

starting position

Sit on the center of the ball. Walk your legs away from the ball and sink the hips so that you are in a squat position. Holding the small ball, make a circle with your arms.

movement: rolling from side to side

1. Inhale to round the arms so that the small ball is in line with the breastbone (fig. 4.86).
2. Exhale. Sink the navel toward the spine and rotate. Keep the same relationship between the small ball and the breastbone (fig. 4.87).
3. Inhale as you rotate back to center.
4. Exhale to rotate to the other side. Keep the same relationship between the small ball and your breastbone. Keep shoulders back and not rounded forward.
5. Repeat six times on each side.

Ball Balance

This exercise will stretch the back of the legs as well as work the abdominals. If there is tightness in the hips or hamstrings, getting the ball in place will be challenging. Use the small ball under the hips to aid you in working against the wall. Once you are up in the position try to lift the ball a couple of inches away from the wall. Balancing the ball on your feet will cause the abdominals to work very hard. In fact, they may work so hard that the superficial rectus muscle bulges out. Place your fingers on or below your navel and check that your abdominals are not pressing into your fingers and popping out. Instead, scoop the navel, hold the contraction of the deep abdominals, and breathe naturally into the back of the ribs. The feet should be apart to allow the ball to balance on the soles.

Purpose To challenge your sense of balance and work the back of the legs and the abdominals.

Watchpoints • Do not rush in or out of the balance. • Be sure that your feet are hip-distance apart and that the ball is balancing on your soles, and not the sides, of your feet. • If you have tight hamstrings you will need to be farther away from the wall.

starting position

Bend your knees as deeply as possible into your chest. Take the ball into your hands. If you have tight hamstrings or a tight low back, tuck a soggy small ball under your hips (fig. 4.88).

movement 1: using the wall

1. Scoot your buttocks two to five inches away from a wall. Bend your knees and place the ball against the wall (fig. 4.89).

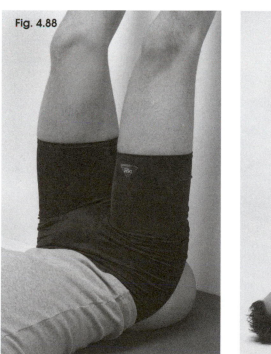

Fig. 4.88

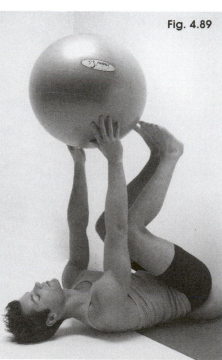

Fig. 4.89

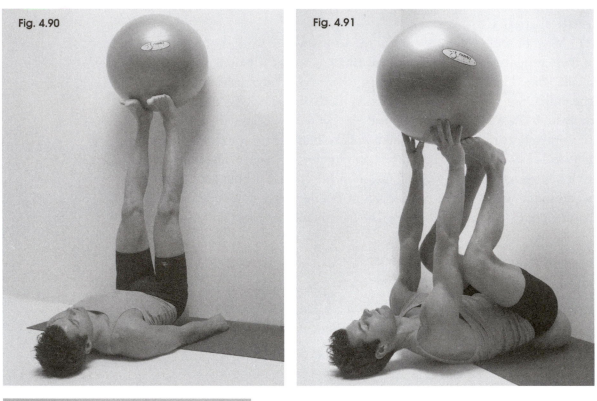

Fig. 4.90

Fig. 4.91

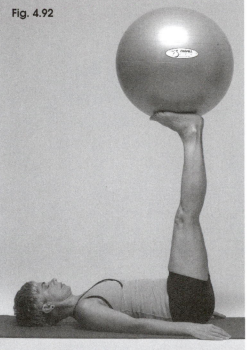

Fig. 4.92

2. Slowly roll the ball up the wall with your feet. Balance the ball as much as you can on the soles, not the sides, of your feet. Your feet should be hip-distance apart (fig. 4.90).

3. Scoop the navel and hold this position for a few breaths.

4. To come out of Ball Balance, slowly bend the legs as deeply as possible, eventually taking the ball into your hands (fig. 4.91).

movement 2: away from the wall

1. Lie on your back with the ball in your hands.

2. Bend the knees into your chest and slowly attempt

to rest the ball on the soles, not the sides, of your feet. Feet should be hip-distance apart.

3. Slowly straighten your legs, keeping the ball balanced on the soles of your feet (fig. 4.92).

4. When the legs are completely straight, hold the balance for as long as you like.

5. Gently tap your abdominals. Make sure they are scooped and not popping out.

6. To come out of Ball Balance, slowly bend the legs, eventually taking the ball into your hands.

7. Roll onto your side and slowly come up.

5

Intermediate
Abs on the Ball

The intermediate work is invigorating and inviting, designed to challenge those who have successfully completed the basic Abs on the Ball exercises and have no limitation or injuries. Breath continues to target the deep abdominals and assist the body to move as efficiently as possible. Ensure quality of movement by infusing each exercise with precision and control; even the most formidable exercise should have an effortless quality. When ready, alter the base of support by taking away points of contact with the mat or the ball and by increasing the length of levers. "Increasing the lever" means extending a limb or limbs away from the axis of rotation, such as the center of the body or shoulder or hip joint, demanding greater effort on the part of the deep core muscles. Changing your orientation to gravity, expanding the range of movement from a small move-ment to its fullest length, and minimizing the base of support will challenge the body and hasten the muscle reeducation process, but only if the core is strong. The inner support must be in place before the movements of outer limbs are added or you will simply be teaching the body a faulty pattern.

As with the last chapter, start with the fundamentals and repeat them often.

Practicing the Fundamentals

The intermediate preliminaries may look simple from the outside. You are not just sitting on a ball or lying on a mat, however, but using the deep core muscles to hold the spine steady and keep the pelvis and body in optimal posture while adding small movements of the limbs. On the in breath expand the rib cage sideways but do not force the inhalation. On the out breath gently draw the navel inward to activate the abdominals. Locating and training the deep transversus abdominis, and then holding the proper contraction for longer and longer periods of time, will build endurance and strength and provide the inner support needed for the challenging exercises to come.

Fundamental #1: Neutral Spine Sitting

Sit tall in the center of your ball and check your posture in a mirror or with your hands. Notice whether the three natural curves of the spine are in place, or whether you are flattening them or exaggerating any of them. A few gentle bounces will activate the correct muscles necessary to align the body in neutral spine. Posner-Mayer explains that when bouncing on a ball "the spine will gravitate to the most comfortable, energy efficient position (optimal posture) by putting the body's center of gravity over its base of support." Abdominal muscles also will work.

Purpose To find the three natural curves of the back (neutral spine).

Watchpoints • When bouncing on the ball keep the head up; don't let the gaze or the head drop. Keep hands touching the ball at first. • Never combine rotation or bending of the spine with bouncing.

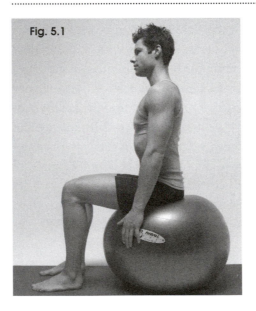

Fig. 5.1

starting position
Sit in the center of your ball, knees aligned with the ankles, legs shoulder-distance apart, feet parallel.

movement 1: bouncing
1. Press your feet to the floor, activate the thighs and calves, and bounce three or four times. Breathe naturally.
2. Stop bouncing. Check your posture in a mirror or with your hands. You should be in neutral spine. There is a curve in the low back, but that curve is not exaggerated. The neck is long but not tense. The ears are aligned over the shoulders (fig. 5.1).

Fundamental #2:
Finding the Core Sitting

Now that you have found neutral spine you will attempt to sit on the ball while holding the deep abdominal connection and resting for ten to twenty-five seconds. Then you will keep the contraction but add small movements of the legs and feet. Closing the eyes alters the awareness of where your body is in space and makes the exercise more difficult. Then try placing the feet on soggy small balls and keeping the trunk and legs stable.

Purpose To train the deep abdominal contraction and control neutral upright posture. Trains nervous system and balance.

Watchpoints • Do not lose optimal posture or neutral pelvis as you lift your toes, close your eyes, or move your feet closer together. Keep your hands on the ball at first. • Watch for changes in posture at the upper chest (with the head poking forward), or changes in the curve of the lower back (an exaggerated curve or flattening). • Sitting and holding the deep contraction is an endurance activity. Start for a short period of time and add time as you get stronger. • Do not hold your breath.

starting position

Sit on the center of the ball, knees aligned with ankles, legs shoulder-distance apart and parallel. Feet are firmly planted, toes long and relaxed. Shoulders are relaxed as you lengthen through the tops of the ears. Chin is level.

movement 1: open eyes

1. Think of gently pulling the navel up and toward the back of the spine. Inhale.
2. Exhale to activate the deep transversus. Think of narrowing the waist, not just flattening it (fig. 5.2).
3. Hold the abdominal connection for 10 to 25 seconds, breathing naturally.
4. Release and rest for10 to 15 seconds.
5. Repeat, holding for 10 to 25 seconds. Do not hold your breath.
6. Release.
7. Repeat the same movement twice with the feet closer together.

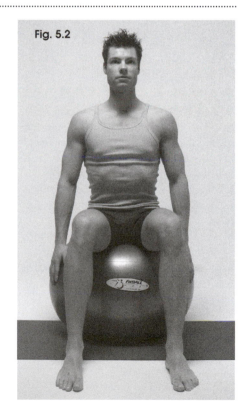
Fig. 5.2

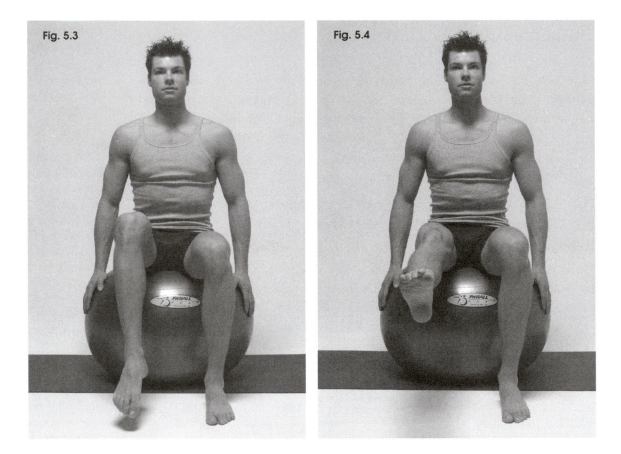

Fig. 5.3   Fig. 5.4

movement 2: eyes closed

1. Start with the feet shoulder-distance apart, hands on the ball. Think of gently pulling the navel up and into the back of the spine. Inhale.

2. Exhale to activate the deep transversus abdominis. Think of narrowing the waist, not just flattening it. Close your eyes.

3. Hold the abdominal contraction for 10 to 25 seconds, breathing naturally.

4. Release and rest for 10 to 25 seconds.

5. Repeat, holding for 10 to 25 seconds. Do not hold your breath.

6. Release.

movement 3: lift toes

1. Inhale to prepare, gently pulling the navel into the spine.

2. Exhale to narrow the waist and lift one foot two inches off the mat (fig. 5.3).

3. Inhale to set the foot down, keeping the abdominal connection.

4. Exhale and lift the other foot two inches.

5. Repeat four times for each leg, keeping the contraction but breathing naturally.

movement 4: lift leg and extend

1. Inhale to prepare, drawing the navel into the spine.

2. Exhale to narrow the waist and extend one leg straight out from the knee (fig. 5.4).

3. Hold steady for a few counts, breathing naturally and keeping the abdominal connection.

4. Set the foot down on the mat and try the other side.

5. Repeat four times with each leg, keeping the contraction but breathing naturally.

movement 5: feet on two small balls

1. Carefully place one foot and then the other on two very deflated small balls (fig. 5.5).

2. Think of pulling the navel up and into the back of the spine. Inhale.

3. Exhale to activate the deep transversus. Think of narrowing the waist, not just flattening it.

4. Try to keep the trunk and legs stable. Breathe naturally and hold the abdominal contraction for as long as you can keep balance.

5. Repeat four times.

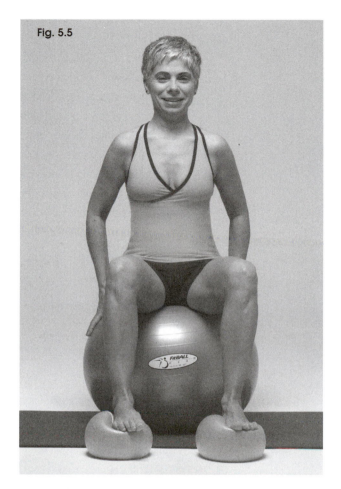

Fig. 5.5

Ball Sitting

*e*xercise ball pioneer and physiotherapist Joanne Posner-Mayer believes that the lack of spinal muscular endurance found in many people today is probably related to how much time people spend in supported sitting. Sitting on a chair, she explains, creates passive support, whereas a ball is a dynamic sitting surface. Sitting on a ball is active—continuous adjustments occur in the body when sitting on a ball. These adjustments train the endurance capacity of the postural muscles and inner core. Physiotherapist and author Rick Jemmett uses ball sitting to help his patients train the deepest layer of the body: the discs, ligaments, and small muscles that run from one vertebra to the next. These are the ligaments and muscles that help stabilize the spinal column and send the brain key information about the position of the joints and bones of the spine. His patients maintain a quality transversus abdominis contraction and keep their balance while adjusting the base of support, opening and closing their eyes, and holding each pose a few seconds longer every day.

Fundamental #3:
Knee Lift Stabilizing Exercise on Small Ball

This is a highly effective way to train the deep transversus abdominis in a very specific manner. Usually Knee Lift is done on the mat, but I find that doing the exercise on a small, slightly soggy ball is a tremendous aid. Here is an example of a small movement that brings results—the ball's instability causes sleepy muscles to fire. After mastering one leg at a time, hold both legs in the air with precision, taking care to keep the contraction while you lift the second knee. Place your fingers one inch in from the hipbones and press in to feel whether you have good control in the transversus abdominis. Remember also to use the drawing in and tightening of the pelvic floor to aid you.

Purpose To find the deep abdominal connection.

Watchpoint • If you no longer feel tension on your fingertips do not raise the leg so high. It is more important to keep the contraction than to lift the knee high.

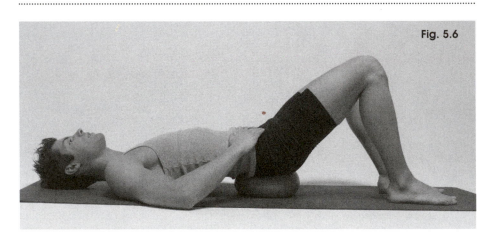

Fig. 5.6

starting position

Lie on your back, lift your knees to your chest, and nestle a slightly deflated small ball under your hips. The small ball will rest under the pelvis, not the low back. Place your feet hip-distance apart on the mat. Head and shoulders are completely relaxed on the mat.

movement 1: single knee lift

1. Place your fingertips one inch in from your hipbones and press in. Inhale to prepare.
2. Exhale to draw in your lower abdomen, pull up the pelvic floor, and find the contraction of the deep transversus abdominis muscle.
3. Inhale to keep the contraction. You should continue to feel tension in your fingertips (fig. 5.6).

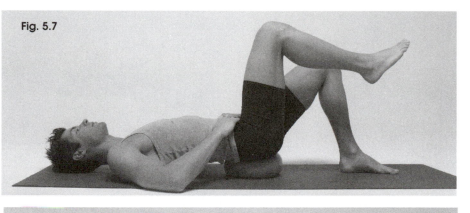

Fig. 5.7

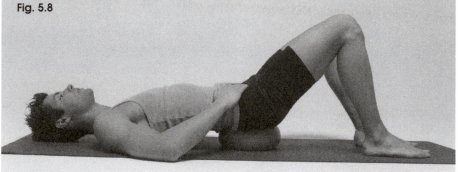

Fig. 5.8

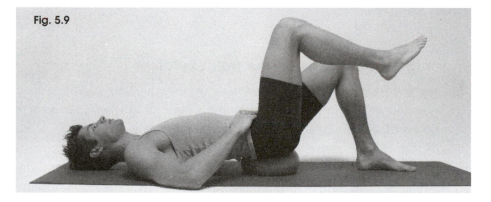

Fig. 5.9

4. Exhale to lift one knee so that the leg is in table-top position (fig. 5.7).
5. Inhale to slowly lower the foot back onto the mat, keeping the abdominal connection.
6. Exhale to lift the other knee to tabletop position.
7. Inhale and place the foot back on the mat.

8. Repeat six times, keeping the abdominal connection.

movement 2: double knee lift

1. Start with both feet on the mat. Inhale to pre-pare (fig. 5.8).
2. Exhale to draw in your lower abdomen, pull up

the pelvic floor, and find the contraction of the transversus.
3. Inhale to keep the con-traction. You should con-tinue to feel tension on your fingertips.
4. Exhale to maintain contraction and lift the right leg to tabletop posi-tion (fig. 5.9).

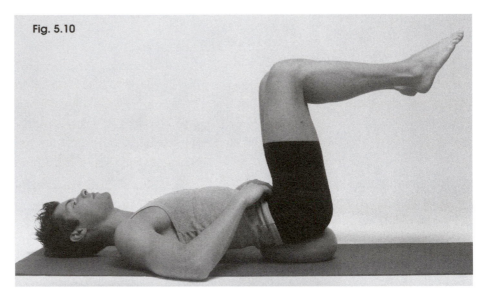

Fig. 5.10

5. Inhale to keep the contraction as you hold the right leg up.
6. Exhale to lift the left leg to join the right in tabletop position (fig. 5.10).
7. Inhale and stay in tabletop legs.

8. Exhale to slowly bring the feet down to the mat.
9. Repeat six to eight times, maintaining the deep abdominal contraction.

The Intermediate Abs on the Ball Exercises

Are you warmed up enough to progress to the intermediate exercises? The fundamentals provide more of a warm-up for your mind than your body—when you feel ready to begin working with the intermediate exercises use the basic fifteen-minute workout at the back of the book or do some gentle aerobic moves to heat up the muscles. Use caution and good sense when working with the larger ball, as there is more potential for injury than when working with the small ball. Work at your own pace.

Full Roll-up

This is a classic Pilates exercise. The ball will add resistance and make your abdominals work very hard. It also heightens your awareness of where your body is in space and adds an element of grace and fun to the exercise. Do not let the ball distract you from rolling your spine like a wheel. Imagine the abdominals are brakes that can slow down the unrolling of the spine. Start with a small ball held in the hands if desired. You can have the legs straight or bent; if they are straight you will feel an invigorating hamstring stretch. You should avoid this exercise if you have low-back pain.

Purpose To strengthen the abdomimals and learn to keep these muscles flat. To experience a hamstring and spine stretch.

Watchpoints • Be sure that the shoulders slide down the back and that you do not arch the upper back off the mat when you take the ball overhead. • Sink the navel toward the spine to roll down one bone at a time. • Flex the feet and push the heels away from the hips to experience a hamstring stretch.

Modification • If you have a tight lower back try bending the knees and keeping the feet far from the buttocks.

....

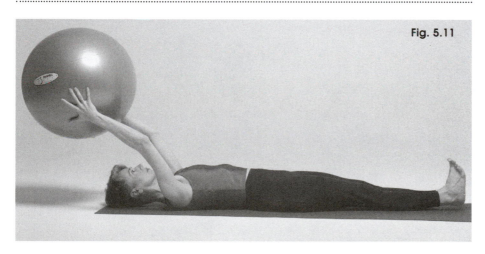

Fig. 5.11

starting position

Lie flat on your back with your legs together, holding the ball between your hands. Keeping your shoulder blades on the mat, take the ball overhead (fig. 5.11). If the knees are bent be sure that the heels are not too close to your buttocks.

why can't I roll up?

Many students are disappointed that they are not able to roll all the way up in exercises like Full Roll-up. Are their abdominals weak? Weak abdominals are not always at issue. Sometimes the physical proportions of the body hamper a student from curling all the way up. Perhaps the legs are short and not heavy enough in comparison to the upper body and trunk, which may be why men in particular often struggle with this exercise. They may need to wrap a thera-band (a wide, five-foot exercise elastic) around their feet or behind their thighs to aid them.

Some students have too much curve in the lower back because tight hip flexors pull the pelvis down in front, preventing them from rolling through the spine. If this is the case for you, try bending the legs, keeping the feet far from the buttocks, and tucking the feet under weights or a strap.

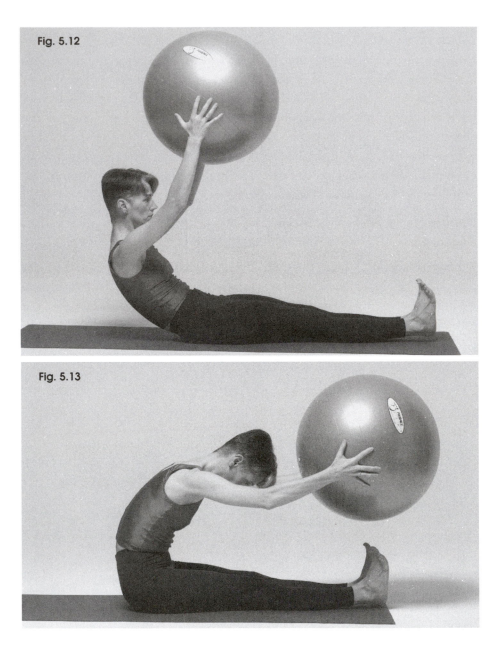

Fig. 5.12

Fig. 5.13

movement: *full roll-up*

1. Inhale to lift the ball to the ceiling.
2. Exhale to flex the body upward, peeling away from the mat one vertebra at a time (fig. 5.12).
3. Inhale to extend the ball toward your toes, then start to roll back, pulling your navel toward your spine (fig. 5.13).

4. Exhale to reverse the movement, rolling down one vertebra at a time.
5. When your shoulder blades reach the mat the ball floats back overhead.
6. Repeat eight times.

Double Leg Stretch

This is a graceful yet powerful Pilates exercise designed to build the power-house. There is a flow and control between the stretching out of the limbs and the tight ball position in between. As with all of these exercises, we are marrying the breath with the movement. Remember, it is the breath that will help relax you and keep you working with the greatest efficiency during the intermediate and advanced exercises. The extra weight of the ball makes this a supreme abdominal tightener, so start with the small ball as support for the body if necessary. Let the small ball support you, but don't collapse into it.

Purpose To build the abdominals and coordination. To practice linking breath with movement.

Watchpoints • Be sure that the arms extend to beside the ears or slightly in front of them, but not behind. • Keep the gaze on the knees, not on the ceiling. • Do not let your legs drop so low that your low back arches off the mat. • Do not hunch the shoulders, and try not to allow the head to poke forward.

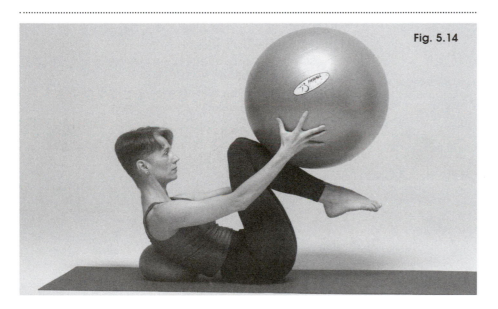

Fig. 5.14

starting position

Place the small ball between the shoulder blades or just below them. Pull your knees into your chest. The low back will drop on the mat. Hold the large ball on your knees or ankles (fig. 5.14).

77

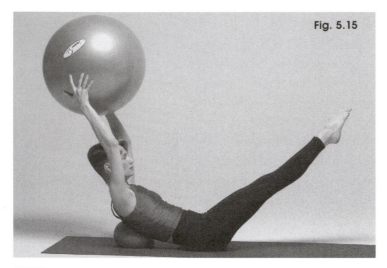

Fig. 5.15

movement 1: with small ball support

1. Inhale to prepare.

2. Exhale to pull the navel toward the spine and extend legs and arms. Arms are just in front of the ears and legs are 45 degrees or higher from the floor (fig. 5.15).

3. Inhale to curl into a ball, bringing the ball to your ankles.

4. Exhale to stretch the legs and arms.

5. Repeat eight times.

movement 2: without small ball support

1. Lying on your back on the mat, pull your knees to your chest.

2. Hold the large ball on your ankles or knees (fig. 5.16).

3. Inhale to lift the head and curl up into a ball (fig. 5.17).

4. Exhale to draw the navel inward and extend the legs and arms. Arms are just in front of the ears, legs 45 degrees or higher from the floor (fig. 5.18).

5. Inhale to curl into a ball, bringing the ball to your ankles.

6. Exhale to stretch the legs and arms.

7. Repeat eight times.

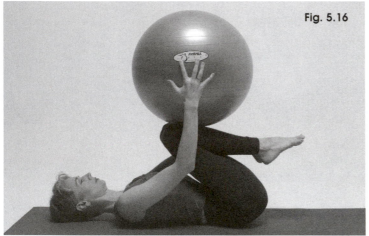

Fig. 5.16

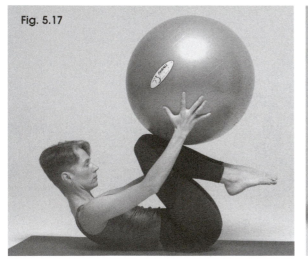

Fig. 5.17

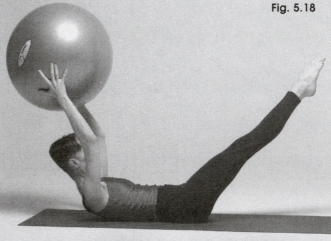

Fig. 5.18

Teaser Prep

This is another superb Pilates abdominal challenge. Here you focus on rolling through the spine one bone at a time as you peel the body off the mat to go up into the air and then return the body to the mat. It is important to work slowly in the peeling up and the lowering down parts of the exercise. Lifting the feet from the ground creates a lever and makes the body work harder to maintain your balance. Squeezing the small ball between the knees keeps the legs in alignment and helps you find the deep abdominal scoop.

Purpose To tone the abdominals and practice articulating through the spine.

Watchpoints • Make sure the feet are not too close to the buttocks to start. • Take care when you lift your arms not to allow the shoulders to raise up to your ears. • Lift from the chest, not the head, as you peel off the mat. Do not pitch yourself upward.

starting position

Lie on your back and place your feet flat on the mat. Place a small ball between your knees. Lift your arms straight above you, ensuring that your shoulder blades remain on the mat (fig. 5.19).

movement 1: feet on the mat

1. Reach your arms back overhead. Use the abdominal connection to ensure that your rib cage is not popping out or that your back is arching (fig. 5.20).
2. Inhale to reach the fingers toward the ceiling.

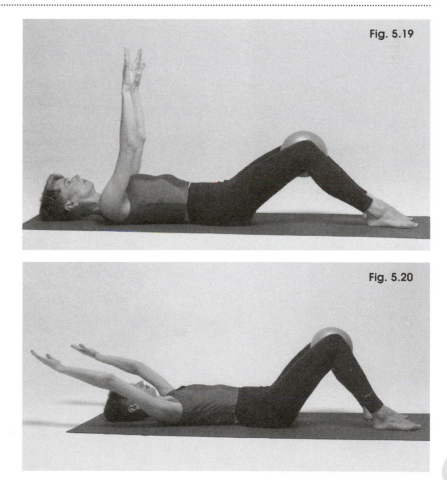

Fig. 5.19

Fig. 5.20

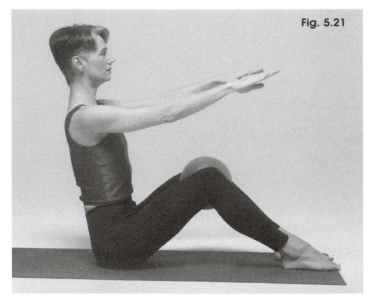

Fig. 5.21

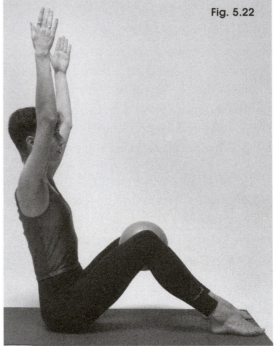

Fig. 5.22

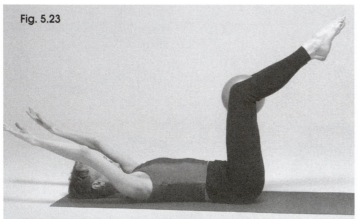

Fig. 5.23

3. Exhale as you scoop your navel toward your spine, press your sacrum into the mat, and continue the movement forward so that your head and upper body follow your hands up in the air (fig. 5.21). You are balancing just behind your sitz bones. The feet should remain planted on the mat.

4. Inhale to lift your arms just in front of the ears. Shoulders remain down (fig. 5.22).

5. Exhale to drop the navel, then roll your spine down to the mat, pressing one bone at a time into the floor.

6. Return to the starting position with arms overhead.

7. Repeat six times.

movement 2: legs in the air

1. The starting position is the same as in movement 1, except the legs are in the air, knees bent. The toes should either be at the same height as the knees or higher. Take the arms slightly back (fig. 5.23).

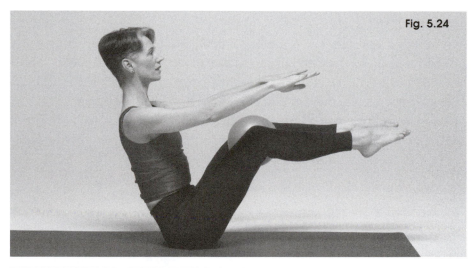

Fig. 5.24

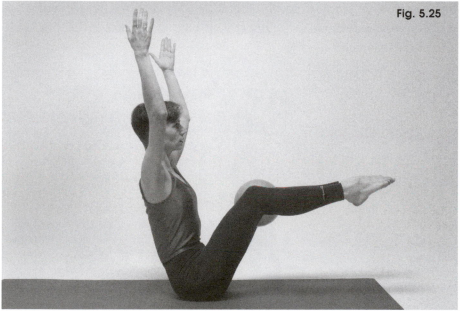

Fig. 5.25

2. Inhale to bring the hands to the ceiling.

3. On the exhale press your sacrum into the mat and continue the movement forward and up so that your head and upper body follow the hands into the air. You are balancing just back of your sitz bones. Ideally the toes are at the same height as the knees or slightly higher (fig. 5.24).

4. Inhale to lift the arms back slightly so that they are just in front of the ears. The shoulders remain down (fig. 5.25). The legs should remain in place.

5. Exhale to drop the navel and roll your spine back down to the mat, pressing one bone at a time into the floor. Keep your knees bent and your feet in the air.

6. Return to the starting position, arms overhead.

7. Repeat six times.

Lower and Lift

This exercise works magic on the low abdominals, but it is essential that the low back remain on the mat. I like to add a ball squeeze to challenge the upper body. Remember to keep the elbows slightly bent to allow for a better squeeze. In movement 2, place the hands in a diamond shape under the buttocks. Deep abdominals must work at all times; if your abdominals bulge you have lost the deep connection. Slowly lower and lift your legs so as not to get into the habit of allowing momentum to aid the exercise.

Purpose To target the low abdominals.

Watchpoints • Do not let the legs lower so far that the low back arches off the mat. • Keep the buttocks from lifting off the mat as you lift the legs.

Modification • If you are not very strong or have tight hamstrings, bend the knees. If you are prone to low-back pain, put the ball to the side and place your hands in a diamond shape under your buttocks to protect the low back. Keep the knees bent.

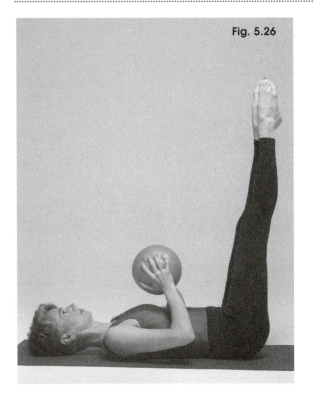

Fig. 5.26

starting position

Lie on your back holding the small ball in front of your chest. Bring your knees to your chest and straighten the legs into the air. Turn the feet out and squeeze the legs together (fig. 5.26).

movement 1: lower and lift

1. Inhale to slowly lower your legs as low as you can while keeping the low back on the mat (fig. 5.27).
2. Exhale to slowly lift the legs. Squeeze the ball on the exhale.
3. Repeat eight times.

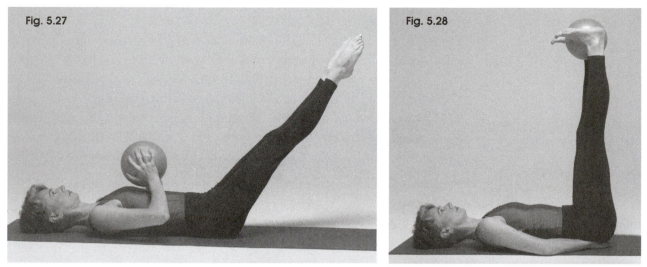

Fig. 5.27

Fig. 5.28

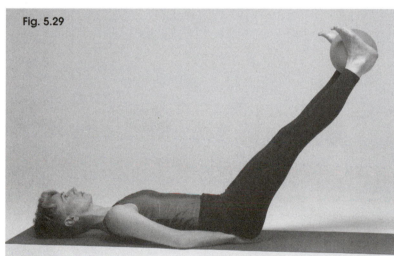

Fig. 5.29

movement 2: small ball between ankles

1. Place a small ball between the ankles and the hands under the buttocks to protect the low back (fig. 5.28).
2. Inhale to lower the legs as low as you can while keeping the low back on the mat (fig. 5.29).
3. Exhale to slowly lift the legs.
4. Repeat eight times.

Do Not Arch the Back off the Mat

*t*he student in this photograph demonstrates an incorrect position as he attempts an intermediate exercise.

Watch for excessive arching of the back in exercises such as Double Leg Stretch and Lower and Lift. Do not let the legs lower so far that the low back arches off the mat. The abdominal and low-back muscles must work in conjunction with each other to stabilize the pelvis.

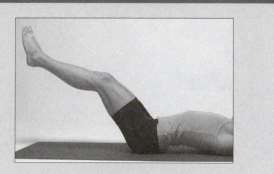

Leg Pull-up and Bicycle

Place the hands in a comfortable position with fingertips facing either forward, sideways, or back. The position of fingers facing forward tends to keep the tension out of the upper trapezius and shoulder muscles, but choose whichever position is comfortable. Leg Pull-up is a Pilates exercise adapted from the matwork. The small ball enables you to take some of the weight out of your wrists. Think of lifting up and off the ball, however, not sinking into it. Glance at your navel from time to time to make sure it is scooped and that the abs are not bulging.

Purpose To tone the abdominals, buttocks, and triceps.

Watchpoints • Keep your hips square and lift the leg only as high as the pelvis remains stable. • Do not sink the pelvis into the ball, as this will place pressure on the knee of the supporting leg. • Hands are underneath the shoulders. • Shoulders are stabilized and not up by the ears.

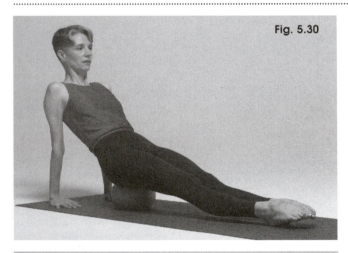

Fig. 5.30

starting position

Sit on the small ball and place the hands directly underneath the shoulders, shifting the weight slightly back. Stretch out your legs, pressing your hips up and tightening your buttocks. Slide your shoulder blades down (fig. 5.30).

movement 1: leg pull-up

1. Inhale and exhale to kick one leg up (fig. 5.31). The toes are long.
2. Inhale to flex the foot and slowly lower the leg, pressing the heel forward (fig. 5.32).
3. At the bottom of the movement exhale as you point the toe, then lift the leg.

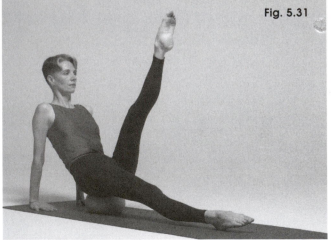

Fig. 5.31

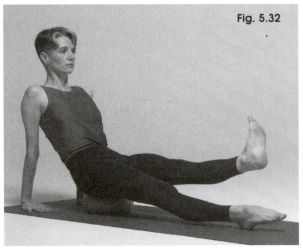

Fig. 5.32

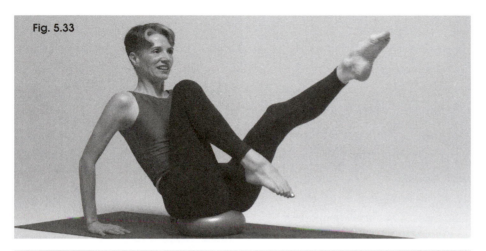

Fig. 5.33

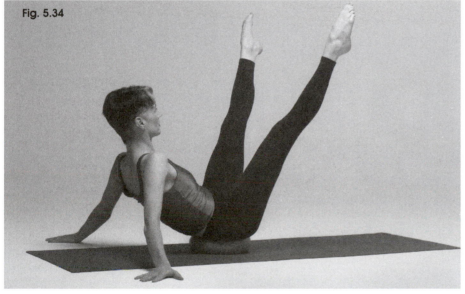

Fig. 5.34

4. Inhale to flex the foot and bring the leg down.

5. Repeat three times with each leg.

movement 2: sitting-on-the-ball bicycle

1. Place your hands on the mat below your shoulders and sit on a small ball. Shift the weight slightly backward into your arms. Bend one leg and then the other, bringing the knees to the chest. Pause until you find your balance.

2. Make a slow and smooth bicycle motion with your legs by circling the legs away from you (fig. 5.33). Breathe naturally.

3. Work for a few counts in one direction, then reverse the direction of the bicycle by pulling the legs toward you.

movement 3: V-shaped legs

1. Change your hand position by opening the fingers to the side and placing the hands wider on the mat. Shift your weight backward. Inhale.

2. Exhale to bend the knees to the chest and straighten both legs into the air.

3. Inhale and open the legs (fig. 5.34).

4. Exhale and close.

5. Repeat six times.

Spine Twist

This is a great abdominal strengthener and spine rotator. Don't forget to squeeze the abdominals as you bring the heavy legs up through center. In movement 2 the extended legs become a longer lever. Increasing the lever makes the deep core muscles work very hard to lift the legs and to stabilize them.

Purpose To challenge and tone the abdominals and inner thighs by adding a longer and longer lever.

Watchpoints • If you have low-back problems keep movement 1 small and avoid movement 2 altogether. • Shoulders and back should remain on the mat throughout the entire exercise.

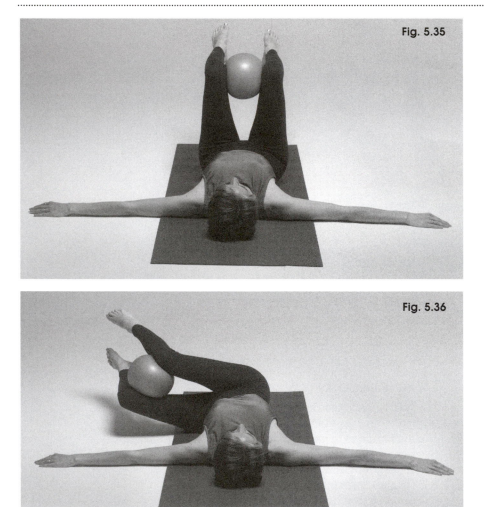

Fig. 5.35

Fig. 5.36

starting position

Lie on the mat with the small ball between the knees. Stretch your arms out to the side in a T shape, palms down.

movement 1: bend knees

1. Gently squeeze the small ball and lift the knees into the air (fig. 5.35).
2. Slowly lower the knees to one side. The knees will not necessarily touch the ground. Keep the shoulders on the mat (fig. 5.36). Breathe naturally through this exercise.
3. Squeeze the abdominals to lift the heavy legs through center.
4. Slowly lower the knees to the other side.
5. Repeat a few times on each side, breathing naturally and moving in your own time.

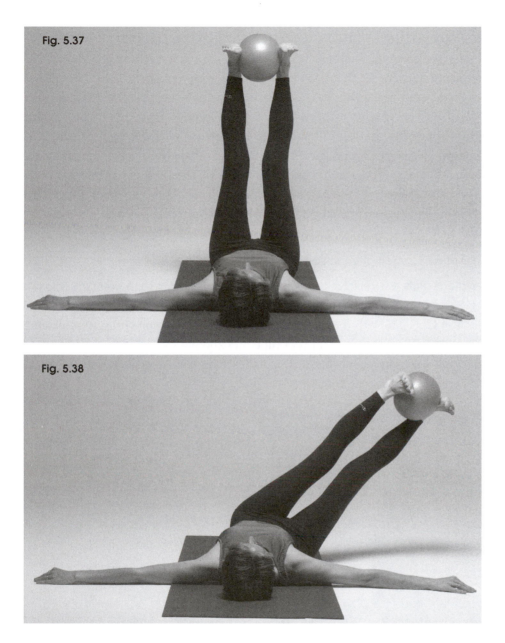

Fig. 5.37

Fig. 5.38

movement 2: straight legs

1. Straighten the legs into the air and squeeze the small ball (fig. 5.37).
2. Slowly lower the legs to one side, keeping the legs straight (fig. 5.38). Keep shoulders on the mat.

3. Hold, then activate the abdominals to lift the legs through the center.
4. Slowly lower the legs to the other side.
5. Repeat a few times on each side, breathing naturally.

Leg Circles, Bicycle, and Scissors in Air

Adapted from the small arc barrel, a Pilates apparatus, these are sensational abdominal exercises that even beginners can do. Remember how as children we used to prop our hips in the air with our elbows and bicycle our legs? The small ball brings this exercise back into everyone's range, even those with tight low backs and tight hamstrings. Resting comfortably under the pelvis, the small ball relieves pressure in the low back and eliminates the urge to roll onto the neck. Note that the small ball rests on the back of the pelvis, not in the curve of the low back; a small portion of the ball may bulge out from under your tailbone when you are in the correct position. It is not necessary to hold the ball in place with your hands—just stretch your fingertips down the mat.

Purpose To strengthen abdominals. To tone the legs and buttocks.

Watchpoints • Don't let the legs circle or open wider than you can control. • Hold the navel-to-spine connection to keep the low back imprinted on the ball. • Check in with the deep transversus muscle from time to time by placing your fingers one inch in from your hipbones and pressing in. • Lopsided leg circles tell you that one side of the deep abdominals may be weaker than the other.

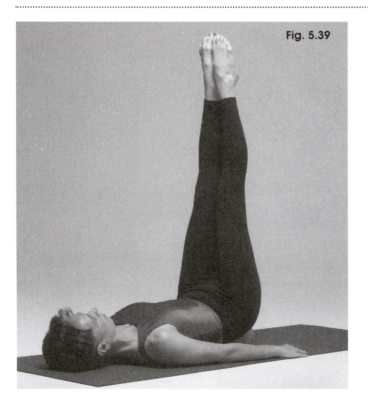

Fig. 5.39

starting position

Lie on the mat and lift your hips slightly to tuck the small ball under your pelvis. Bring your bent knees up toward your chest. Let your weight sink into the ball. Your neck should be relaxed; you should feel no pressure on it.

movement 1: open and close

1. Straighten your legs into the air, toes long. Gently draw the navel toward the spine (fig. 5.39).

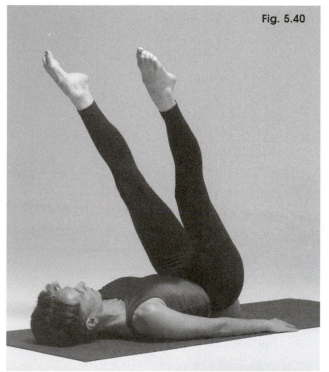

Fig. 5.40

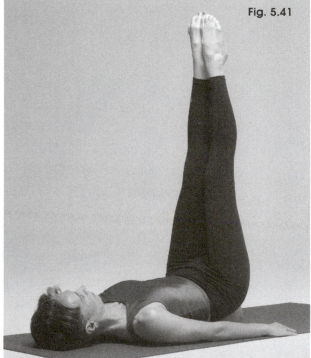

Fig. 5.41

2. Inhale to open your legs shoulder-distance apart (fig. 5.40).

3. Exhale to squeeze your legs closed.

4. Repeat eight times.

movement 2: leg circles

1. Straighten your legs into the air, toes long. Gently draw the navel toward the spine (fig. 5.41).

2. Inhale to bring your legs closer to your head, keeping the legs straight.

3. Exhale to circle the legs around (fig. 5.42).

4. Repeat five times, then reverse the direction of the circle.

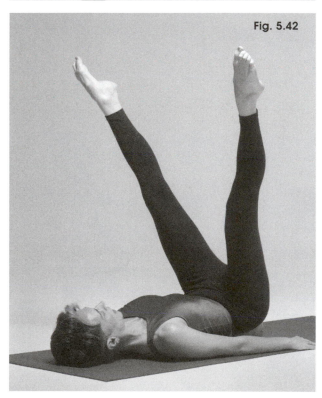

Fig. 5.42

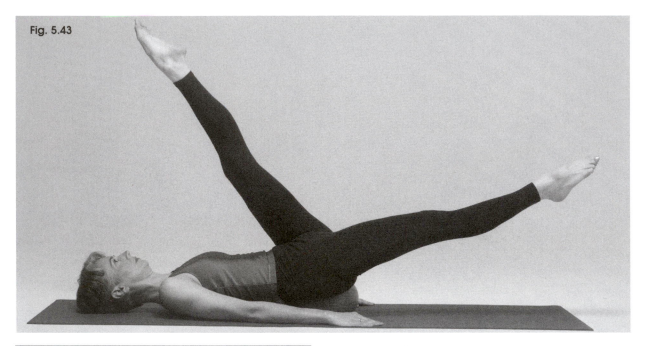

Fig. 5.43

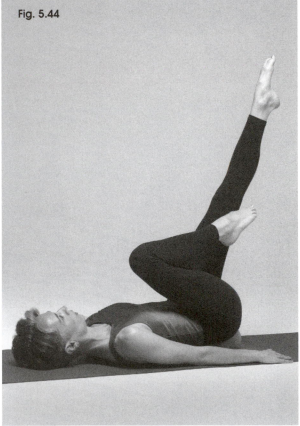

Fig. 5.44

movement 3: scissors in air

1. Straighten your legs into the air, toes long. Gently draw the navel toward the spine.

2. Inhale to prepare.

3. Exhale to reach the left leg up to the ceiling while the right leg lengthens down to the mat (fig. 5.43). Pulse legs twice on the exhale.

4. Inhale to switch legs.

5. Exhale to reach the right leg toward the ceiling while the left leg lengthens down to the mat. Pulse legs twice on the exhale.

6. Inhale to switch legs.

7. Working the right and left side is one set. Repeat six times.

movement 4: bicycle in air

1. Straighten your legs into the air, toes long. Gently draw the navel toward the spine.

2. Breathing naturally, draw one leg down and begin moving your legs in a bicycling motion (fig. 5.44).

3. Turn the bicycle wheel slowly and smoothly five times in one direction.

4. Reverse the rotation of the wheel for five spins. Breathe naturally.

5. To come out of this exercise bend your knees, roll onto your side, and wiggle the small ball out from underneath you.

On Elbows

Talk about discovering forgotten or sleepy muscles! In this exercise the legs move slowly and smoothly and are maintained by the core. Usually this exercise is performed on the mat, but the instability of a small ball forces the inner layer to do its job. If you are not strong enough in the shoulders, however, this exercise may strain your neck. For movement 3 use a 45-cm or soggy 55-cm ball and try not to sink between your shoulders for any of the movements. Keep the knees bent and simply balance if extending the legs is too difficult.

Purpose To keep a strong, stable core while adding smooth and precise movements of the legs.

Watchpoints • Keep the deep abdominals contracted throughout the exercise. • Do not sink between your shoulders. Let your elbows or hands be a strong point of support on the floor.

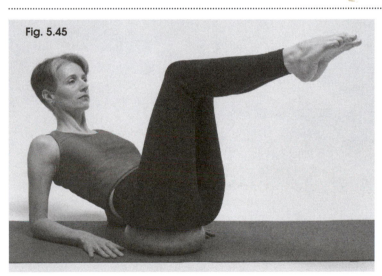

Fig. 5.45

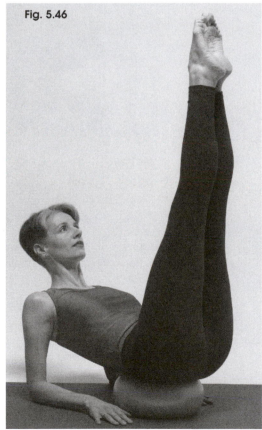

Fig. 5.46

starting position

Lie back on your small ball, setting the pelvis on the ball. Rest the elbows on the mat. Try not to sink the shoulders. Both feet rest on the mat.

movement 1: bend and stretch legs

1. Inhale to prepare. Exhale to pull in your lower abdomen and lift your toes off the mat (fig. 5.45).
2. Inhale and stay.
3. Exhale to straighten both legs into the air (fig. 5.46).
4. Inhale to bend the legs.
5. Repeat six to eight times maintaining the deep transversus contraction.

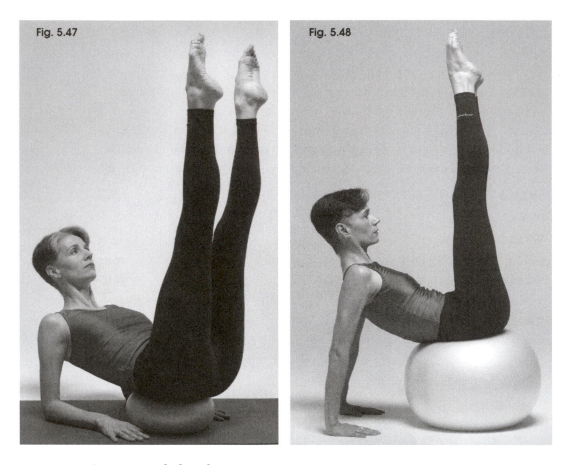

Fig. 5.47

Fig. 5.48

movement 2: open and close legs

1. Inhale to prepare. Exhale to pull in your lower abdomen and lift your toes off the mat.
2. Inhale to open the legs shoulder-distance apart (fig. 5.47).
3. Exhale to squeeze the legs together.
4. Repeat six to eight times maintaining the deep transversus contraction.

movement 3: on hands

1. Sit on a 45-cm or a soggy 55-cm ball. Walk your feet away from the ball and roll through the back until you can place your hands on the mat underneath your shoulders with the fingertips facing forward, sideways, or backward. The low back is on the ball and your weight is on the hands. Shoulders are down.
2. Secure the navel-to-spine connection as you bring one leg and then the other to tabletop position. Steady yourself here. Inhale.
3. Exhale to straighten both legs into the air (fig. 5.48).
4. Inhale to bend. Exhale to extend.
5. Repeat six times.

Thigh and Ankle Squeeze and Supported Swan

For this exercise we roll on to the belly to stretch out the front of the body. Squeezing the small ball between the thighs and ankles works different muscles of the legs and buttocks. In movements 1 and 2 try to keep the buttocks relaxed as you focus on isolating just the inner thigh and pelvic floor muscles. In movements 3 and 4 the buttocks will work. In the Supported Swan do not think of arching up; focus instead on elongating the spine. Pull the navel into the spine and use the deep stabilizing muscles to keep the pelvis level. Think of sending the tailbone away from the hips.

Purpose To tone the abdominals, spinal muscles, inner thighs, and back of legs.

Watchpoints • Keep length in the back of the neck and spine. • Relax your shoulder blades down your back. • In the Supported Swan keep your elbows soft, not hyperextended. Make sure the navel-to-spine connection is secure to protect the low back.

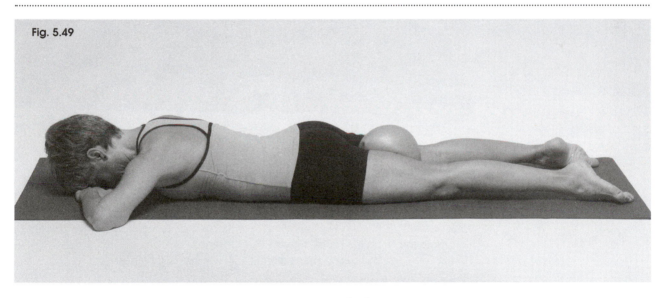

Fig. 5.49

starting position

Lie on your belly. Placing one hand on top of the other, rest your forehead on your hand. Legs are extended on the mat and slightly turned out, hip-distance apart. Toes are long.

movement 1: thigh squeeze

1. Place the small ball between your thighs. Inhale to prepare.
2. Exhale to pull up the navel, tighten the pelvic floor, and gently squeeze the ball between the thighs (fig. 5.49).
3. Inhale to release and exhale to squeeze.
4. Repeat eight times.

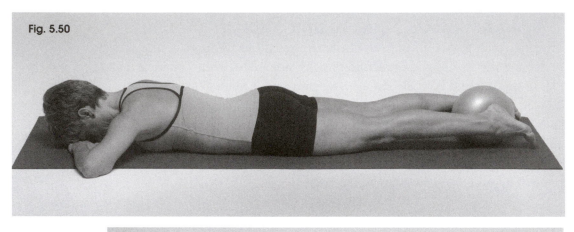

Fig. 5.50

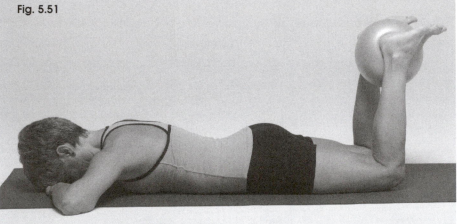

Fig. 5.51

movement 2: squeeze ball at ankles

1. Place the small ball between the ankles.
2. Exhale to pull up the navel, tighten the pelvic floor, and gently squeeze the ball (fig. 5.50).
3. Inhale to release and exhale to squeeze.
4. Repeat eight times.

movement 3: lift ball and squeeze

1. Place the small ball between the ankles. Inhale as you lengthen the legs away from you.
2. Exhale to secure the navel-to-spine connection and tighten the pelvic floor

as you squeeze and lift the ball two inches.
3. Inhale to release and lower the ball to the mat. Exhale to squeeze and lift the ball.
4. Repeat eight times.

movement 4: bend knees and squeeze

1. Place the small ball between the ankles. Inhale.
2. Exhale to lift the navel and lengthen the legs away from you, bending the knees.
3. Keeping the legs bent, inhale to release and exhale to tighten the pelvic floor and squeeze the ball (fig. 5.51).
4. Repeat eight times.

movement 5: supported swan

1. Move the ball to the breastbone. Hands are slightly in front of the shoulders; elbows are on the mat and parallel to the body. Keep the head aligned with the spine but dropped slightly. Your gaze is on the mat (fig. 5.52).

2. Inhale to glide the shoulders downward.

3. Exhale to lift the navel inward and extend the spine upward. Stretch the arms slightly but keep the elbows soft as you elongate the spine (fig. 5.53).

4. Inhale to stay at the top. The gaze is straight ahead.

5. Exhale to return to the starting position. Relax your head.

6. Repeat five times.

movement 6: the cat

1. Rise up to your hands and knees. Your weight should be equally distributed on all four limbs, hands below shoulders and knees below hips. Start in a flat-back position.

2. Inhale to prepare.

3. Exhale to pull up the navel and round the back. The head drops (fig. 5.54).

4. Inhale to return to the flat-back position.

5. Repeat five times.

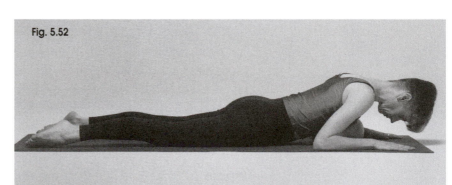

Fig. 5.52

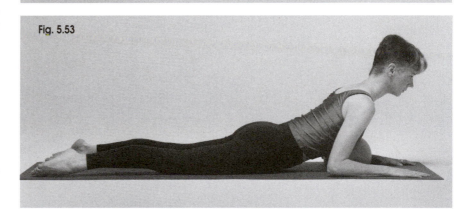

Fig. 5.53

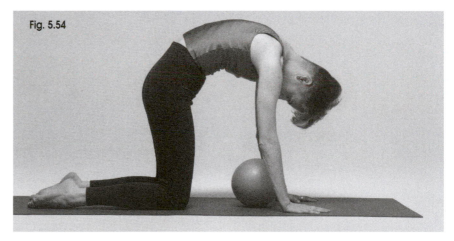

Fig. 5.54

Bend and Stretch

The abdominals work hard in this exercise, but so do the inner and outer thighs. On the exhalation sink the abdominals as you extend the legs. The farther the legs extend the harder the abdominals are working. Hold the deep contraction to keep the pelvis steady and keep the low back from arching. If you have low-back discomfort, keep the legs high in the air and use the small ball.

Purpose To tone the abdominals, legs, hip adductor muscles, and inner thighs.

Watchpoint • Try not to let the body sink between the shoulders. Maintain stability in the abdominals.

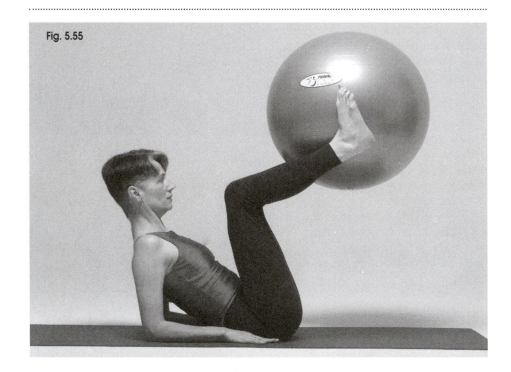

Fig. 5.55

starting position

Rest on your sacrum with your knees bent. Pick up the ball between your ankles and squeeze. Bend the knees inward. Make a strong support with your elbows and don't let the neck sink between the shoulders (fig. 5.55).

movement 1: bend and stretch

1. Inhale to prepare.
2. Exhale as you extend the legs 45 degrees or higher from the floor (fig. 5.56).
3. Inhale to draw the ball toward you.
4. Exhale to extend the legs.
5. Perform this exercise six to eight times.

movement 2: with ball twist

1. Extend the legs 45 degrees or higher from the floor.
2. Keeping the legs straight, swivel the ball from side to side and breathe naturally (fig. 5.57).

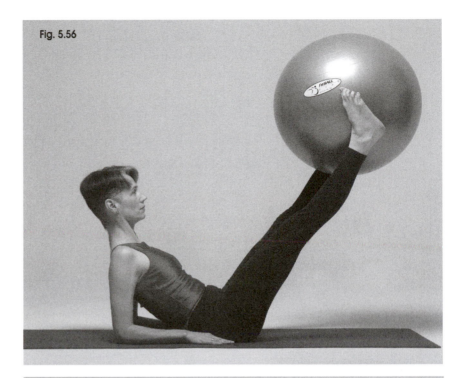

Fig. 5.56

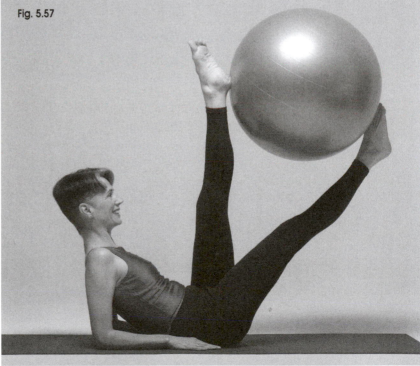

Fig. 5.57

Backward Crunch

This is a very effective exercise that targets the low abdominals. You will be hugging the large ball with the back of the legs and then lifting the legs toward the chest. As you raise the hips slightly off the mat, keep the low back pressed down.

Purpose Strengthens the low abdominals and the hamstrings.

Watchpoints • Keep the low back pressed to the floor as you bring your knees up and back. • Try to keep the shoulders, neck, and jaw relaxed.

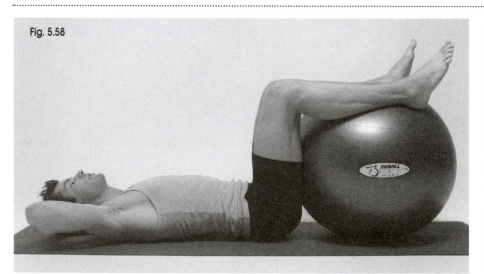

Fig. 5.58

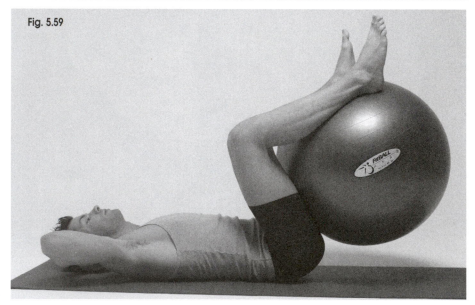

Fig. 5.59

starting position

Lie on your back, bend your knees, and squeeze a large ball with the back of your thighs and heels. Place your hands behind your head or stretch them down beside the body (fig. 5.58).

movement 1: backward crunch

1. Inhale to prepare.
2. Exhale to bring the knees in toward your chest, slowly raising the hips off the floor (fig. 5.59).
3. Inhale and stay.
4. Exhale to release back to the mat.
5. Repeat eight times.

Hip Lift

You will feel this exercise in the back of the legs, the hamstrings, and the buttocks as well as in the deep core muscles. Do not arch the back and make sure your navel-to-spine connection is secure. Start small and feel the deep centering muscles, including the pelvic floor, working together to keep the spine and pelvis steady. For a real challenge to the core try this exercise with the feet on the small ball. When you lower the torso back to the mat do so with control, one vertebra at a time.

Purpose To challenge the abdominal core and balance, and to work the back of the legs, the hamstrings, and the buttocks.

Watchpoints • Keep knees close together in the Hip Lift. • Do not push the hips up too high. • Stay relaxed through the back of the neck, the jaw, and the shoulders. • Keep equal pressure in both feet.

starting position

Lie on your back with your knees bent and the soles of your feet on a large ball.

movement 1: hip lift on large ball

1. Inhale to press your feet into the ball.
2. Exhale to curl the tailbone and sequence up one bone at a time until the knees, hips, and shoulders are in a straight line (fig. 5.60).
3. Inhale to stay at the top of the movement for a few breaths. Hold steady.
4. Exhale to sequence slowly back to the mat.
5. Repeat five times.

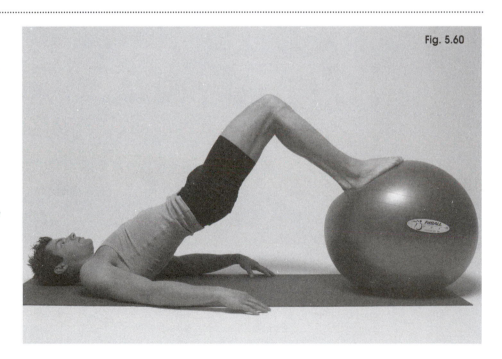

Fig. 5.60

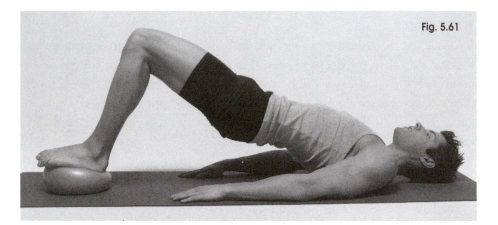

Fig. 5.61

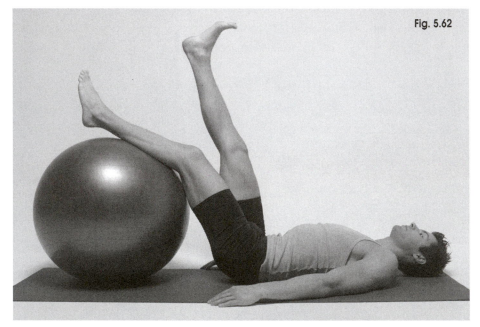

Fig. 5.62

movement 2: on small ball

1. Inhale to press your feet into a small ball.
2. Exhale to curl the tailbone and sequence up one bone at a time until the knees, hips, and shoulders are in a straight line (fig. 5.61).
3. Inhale to stay at the top of the movement for a few breaths. Hold steady.
4. Exhale to sequence slowly back to the mat.
5. Repeat five times.

movement 3: stretch hamstrings

1. Place both calves on the large ball.
2. Lift one leg off the ball, keeping the leg as straight as possible. The back of the knee can be soft. Try to keep the tailbone on the mat (fig. 5.62).
3. Hold for 20 seconds, breathing naturally.
4. Lower the leg to the ball and switch sides.

Back Extensions on Knees

This exercise strengthens the core and the entire back. Remember to pull in the navel before you lift. Work slowly and evenly at a height that is good for your body.

Purpose To strengthen the back and the abdominal muscles.

Watchpoints • Avoid arching the back. • Keep your head in line with your body; keep your upper arms and elbows wide. • Keep shoulders down when the hands are placed on the forehead.

starting position

Kneel in front of your ball and place your belly and rib cage on the ball. Your upper back is parallel with the floor. Hands are placed on the forehead; elbows are wide (fig. 5.63).

movement 1: on knees

1. Inhale to pull in the navel and lift the upper back (fig. 5.64).
2. Exhale to lower the body.
3. Repeat eight times.

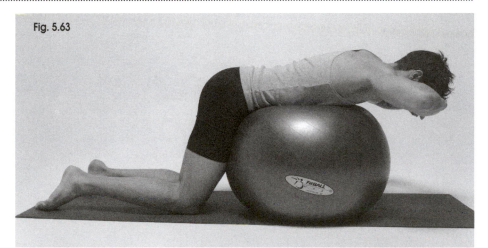
Fig. 5.63

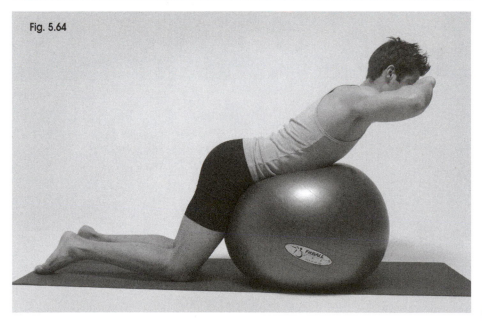
Fig. 5.64

Side Raises

Your body is "stiff as a board" as you lift up in this exercise. Keep the hands on the forehead or the side of the head and the elbows wide. This exercise can also be done kneeling on one knee with the top leg straight out to the side.

Purpose To strengthen the core, the quadratus lumborum, and the obliques.

Watchpoints • Keep the abdominals connected. • Avoid arching your back or letting your waist sag toward the ball. • Stay relaxed through the neck, shoulders, and jaw. • Keep the head aligned on the spine.

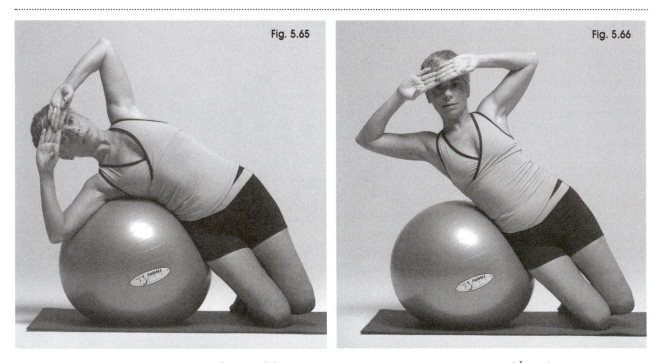

Fig. 5.65   Fig. 5.66

starting position

Kneel next to the ball. Place your side against the ball. Hands are on the forehead.

movement: side raises

1. Press the side of your body against the ball (fig. 5.65).
2. Exhale to lift your body, keeping your body very strong (fig. 5.66).
3. Inhale to return.
4. Do eight repetitions, then repeat on the other side.

Side Crunches

You may well feel soreness the day after performing this exercise. Use a wall to stabilize your feet. Start with the arms folded over your chest and then progress to hands on the forehead. Make sure you lengthen back fully to the ball so that the side muscles can stretch.

Purpose To strengthen the core, the quadratus lumborum, and the obliques.

Watchpoints • Keep your body aligned, hips square. • Stay relaxed through the shoulders, neck, and jaw.

starting position

Place the ball three feet from the wall. Cross your legs so that the bottom foot is in front of the top one. Anchor your feet against the wall. Place your hips on the side of the ball.

movement 1: hands across chest

1. Inhale to lengthen the body sideways across the ball (fig. 5.67).
2. Exhale to pull in the navel and curl up sideways until the hips, knees, and shoulders are in one line (fig. 5.68).
3. Inhale to return the body to the ball.
4. Exhale to curl up sideways.
5. Repeat eight times, then move the ball to the other side.

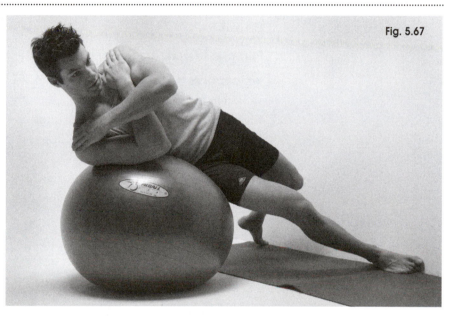

Fig. 5.67

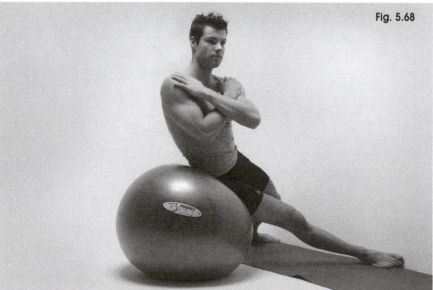

Fig. 5.68

103

Planks

Walking your hands out into a strong Plank with the ball at the shins or ankles is very challenging for the core and the entire body. If you can't maintain the deep abdominal connection don't walk too far: start with the ball on the thighs. The deep abdominals must be engaged to protect the low back and to keep the body from sagging in the middle. The gluteals will also be working: if you turn the legs slightly out from the hip sockets you will be able to connect and tighten the buttocks. Lifting one leg off the ball or taking it to the side is a real balance challenge. The most difficult part of this exercise, however, may be walking the body back toward the ball after you have held the Plank for a few seconds.

Purpose To work the inner core and the entire body, and to practice balance.

Watchpoints • Maintain good stability in the shoulder girdle. • Keep your shoulder blades open and down, not lifted toward the ears. • Elbows are slightly soft, not locked or hyperextended. • Do not let the head drop: keep it in line with the spine. • When lifting the leg off the ball keep the movement small.

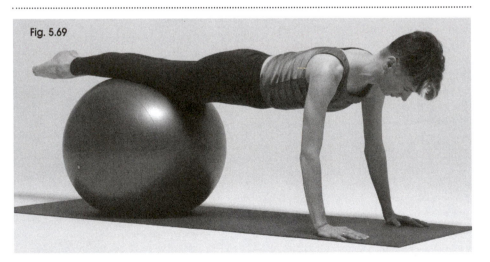

Fig. 5.69

starting position
Kneel in front of the ball. Place hands palm down on the floor.

movement 1: both feet on the ball

1. Walk out until the ball is on the thighs, shins, or ankles, keeping hands just wider than the shoulders. Fingertips should be parallel to the body, elbows angled slightly back. Do not let the midline drop. Keep the legs very straight, and keep the buttocks working (fig. 5.69).

2. Hold this position for a few seconds and breathe naturally.

3. Return by walking the hands back toward the ball.

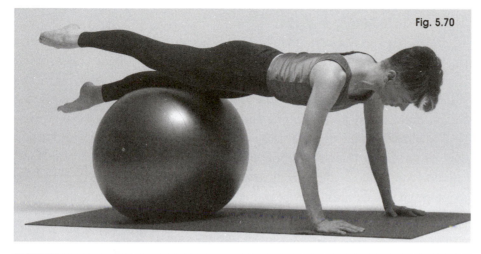

Fig. 5.70

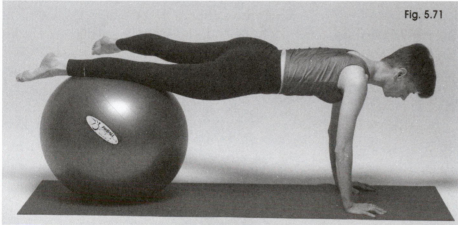

Fig. 5.71

In exercises like Planks and Push-ups, where we take weight on the arms, we need to focus especially on stabilizing the shoulders blades. If we don't do this the muscles around the neck and upper shoulders will overwork. When we take force onto the arms the shoulder blades need to stay tight against the rib cage. Try to keep the shoulder blades from winging, or protruding. The trapezius muscle of the back, other scapular stabilizers (muscles between the shoulder blades), and serratus anterior (a muscle that covers the side of the rib cage, under the armpits) work together to fix the scapulae. Be aware of your shoulders at all times, not just in weight-bearing exercises.

movement 2: lift one foot

1. Walk out until the ball is on the thighs, shins, or ankles, keeping hands just wider than the shoulders. Fingertips should be parallel to the body, elbows angled slightly back. Do not let the midline drop. Keep the legs very straight, and keep the buttocks working.
2. Breathe naturally as you lift one leg a few inches. Keep this leg very straight (fig. 5.70).
3. Place the leg back on the ball. Get centered. Then lift the other leg off the ball and hold. Place it back on the ball.
4. Return by walking the hands back toward the ball.

movement 3: lift foot to side

1. Walk out until the ball is on the thighs, shins, or ankles, keeping hands just wider than the shoulders. Fingertips should be parallel to the body, elbows angled slightly back. Do not let the midline drop. Keep legs very straight, and keep the buttocks working.
2. Breathe naturally as you lift one leg and take it to the side. Keep this leg very straight (fig. 5.71).
3. Place the leg back on the ball. Get centered. Lift the other leg slightly to the side and hold. Place it back on the ball.
4. Return by walking the hands back toward the ball.

Side Shell with Kick

You might choose not to do Planks, Side Shell with Kick, and Arabesque on the same day, because they are all strenuous for the upper body and wrists. It is essential for Side Shell with Kick that the ball is in the correct place. The ball cannot be on the pelvis or the shins; it must be on the bottom of the thighs, immediately in front of the knees. Posner-Mayer calls this exercise the "Prone Skier" because it imitates the movement of the hips, knees, and shoulders on a ski slope. She notes how strenuous this exercise is on the abdominals and the shoulder girdle, as those areas "maintain balance while absorbing momentum." I take this exercise one step further by adding a side kick to it.

Purpose To strengthen the inner core, the abdominal obliques, and the upper body.

Watchpoints • Keep your upper torso square to the ground. • Do not sag in the midriff when you return to Plank position. • Use the abdominals to lift the hips and swivel them to the side.

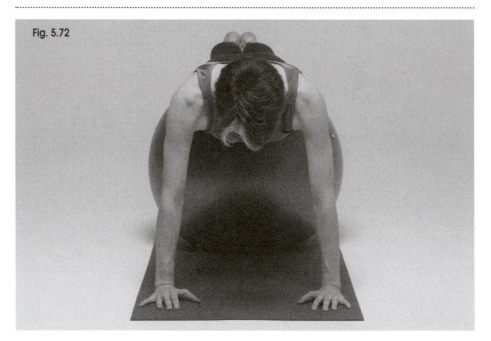

Fig. 5.72

starting position

Kneel in front of your ball. Crawl over the ball and walk out so that the hands are directly below the shoulders and the ball is directly in front of the knees on the thighs. Squeeze thighs together and keep the sides of the knees touching each other (fig. 5.72).

movement 1: without kick

1. Inhale to lengthen through the spine in Plank position.

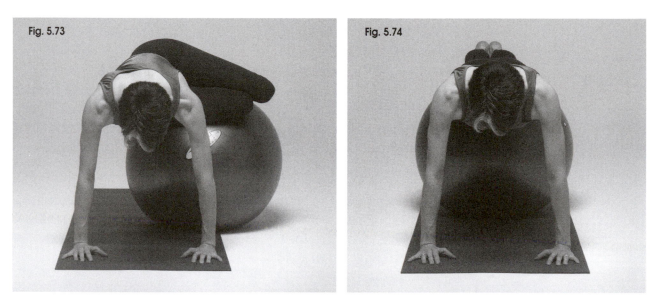

Fig. 5.73

Fig. 5.74

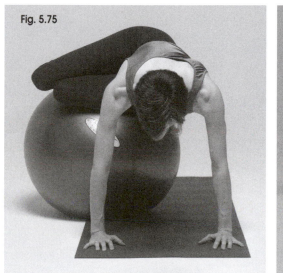

Fig. 5.75

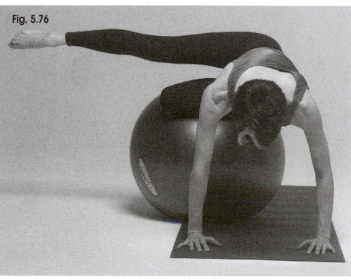

Fig. 5.76

2. Exhale to scoop the navel and bend the knees and hips, swiveling to one side so that the ball comes to the side of the hip (fig. 5.73). Leave the hands firmly planted where they are on the mat.

3. Inhale to stay in Side Shell.

4. Exhale as you take the body straight back to Plank position (fig. 5.74). Make sure you keep the ball controlled as you do this. The ball will roll back into place.

5. Repeat three or four times, alternating sides.

movement 2: with kick

1. Inhale to lengthen through the spine in Plank position.

2. Exhale to scoop the navel and bend the knees and hips, swiveling to one side so the ball comes to the side of the hip (fig. 5.75). Leave the hands firmly planted where they are on the mat.

3. Inhale to extend one leg directly to the side (fig. 5.76).

4. Exhale to bring the knee of that leg back to meet the other knee, controlling the ball as you take the body straight back to Plank position. The ball will roll back into place.

5. Repeat on the other side.

6. Perform three or four repetitions of the exercise, alternating sides.

Arabesque

We approach this tricky balance exercise by first practicing the Stork position, in which you simply lift one knee two inches off the ball. Practice that a few times before lifting the leg straight up in the air. Approach the Side Arabesque not from Plank position but from the side of the ball. Roll your trunk sideways until the ball is under your side rib cage and your hands are on the mat. As the legs lift in the air the upper body pitches slightly forward.

Purpose To strengthen the inner core and practice balance and coordination.

Watchpoints • Do not sag in the midriff when you return to Plank position. • Keep your shoulder blades sliding down • When you lift the leg in movements 1 and 2 try to keep the hips squared. In movement 3 work slowly and cautiously as you roll into position.

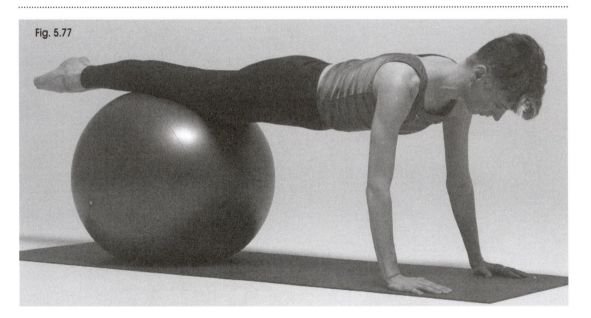

Fig. 5.77

starting position

Kneel in front of your ball. Crawl over the ball and walk out on your hands so that the hands are directly below the shoulders and the ball is directly in front of the knees. Squeeze the thighs together and keep the sides of the knees touching each other.

movement 1: the stork

1. Inhale to lengthen through the spine in Plank position (fig. 5.77).

2. Exhale to bend the knees and hips and let the ball roll under you, leaving the hands firmly planted where they are on the mat. This is the Shell on the Ball position (fig. 5.78).
3. Inhale to lift your tailbone and roll the ball out a couple of inches.
4. Exhale to bend the right knee and lift the right leg slightly; the right heel comes to right buttock (fig. 5.79).

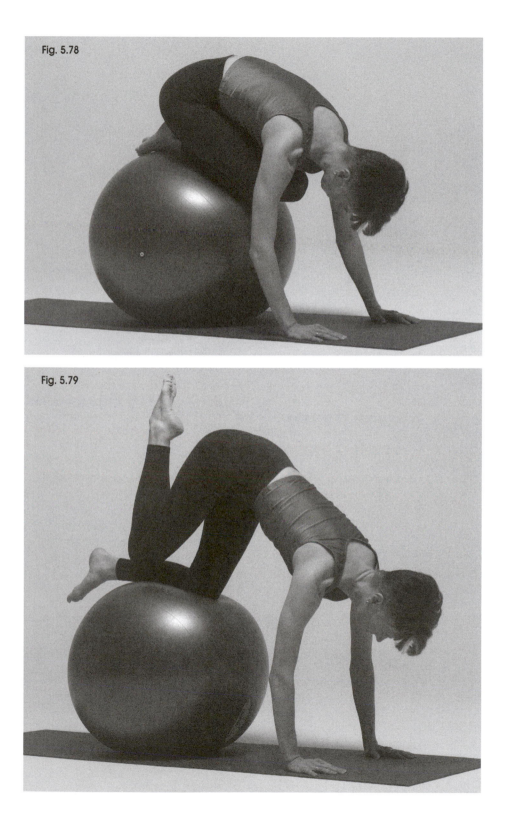

Fig. 5.78

Fig. 5.79

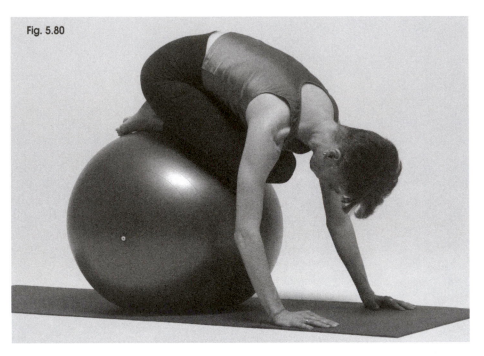

Fig. 5.80

5. Balance for a moment here, breathing naturally.

6. The right knee meets the left knee back on the ball. Return to Shell on the Ball and take a few resting breaths (fig. 5.80).

7. Repeat on the other side, then roll the ball out into Plank position. Walk the hands back to the ball and return to the mat.

movement 2: the arabesque

1. Begin the same way as the Stork, by taking the body into the Shell on the Ball position (fig. 5.80).

2. Inhale to lift your tailbone and roll the ball out a couple of inches.

3. Exhale to bent knee and then lift the right leg and extend it into the air. The leg should be straight, toes long (fig. 5.81).

4. Balance here for a moment, breathing naturally.

5. The right knee meets the left knee back on the ball. Return to Shell on the Ball and take a few resting breaths (fig. 5.82).

6. Repeat on the other side, then roll the ball out into Plank position. Walk the hands back to the ball to return to the mat.

movement 3: side arabesque

1. Place the side of the right hip on the top center of the ball. Your left arm rests on the left thigh (fig. 5.83).

2. Inhale to roll the trunk sideways across the ball until your right hand is slightly behind your shoulder on the mat.

3. Exhale to place the left hand on the mat and lift the legs into the air. The right foot draws to the left knee as the upper body pitches slightly forward and the elbows bend. The head turns in the direction of the legs (fig. 5.84).

4. Inhale and stay. Exhale to roll back in the opposite direction to the starting position.

5. Repeat three times and change sides.

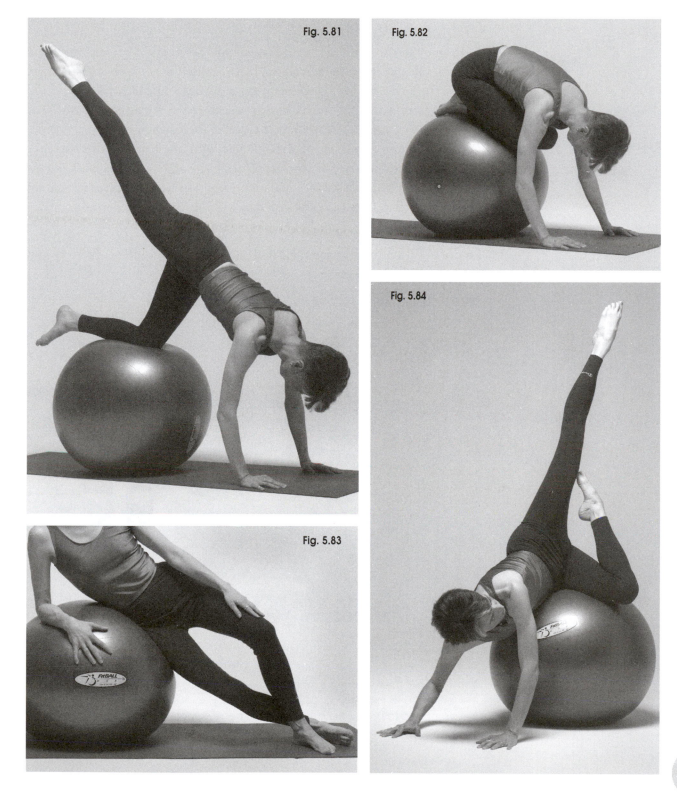

Fig. 5.81

Fig. 5.82

Fig. 5.84

Fig. 5.83

Tabletop Balance

Just something as simple as lifting one toe off the ground without letting the ball roll out shows the belly working hard—sometimes it will even tremble. Pull in the navel, narrow the waist, and use the deep core muscles to hold you upright. Start by holding the floor with your fingertips for assistance with balance. Eventually move the feet closer together for a greater challenge. Joanne Posner-Mayer proposes writing the alphabet with one lifted foot in exercises such as Tabletop Balance or Planks. "Writing the alphabet adds random perturbations to challenge balance and proprioception while adding momentum and inertia." She suggests increasing speed and the size of the letters for extra challenge.

Purpose To tone the abdominals and other spinal stabilizers. To work the gluteals and back of legs.

Watchpoints • Keep hips up and straight as a board. • Do not let your mid-section sag. • Keeping the pelvis lifted and stable is more important than how high you lift the leg.

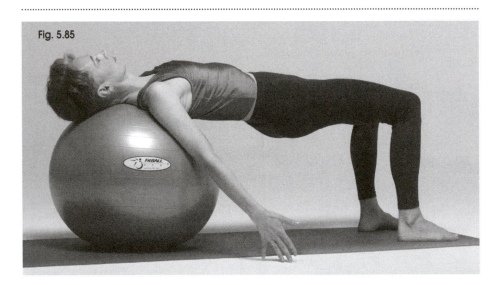

Fig. 5.85

starting position

Sit on the ball, then lean back and walk the feet out until the head and neck are supported totally by the ball. You can touch the ground for assistance with balance.

movement: tabletop balance

1. Inhale to prepare in Tabletop position. Hands should be either behind the head or loosely touching the ground (fig. 5.85).

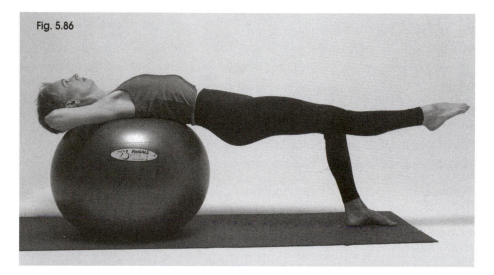

Fig. 5.86

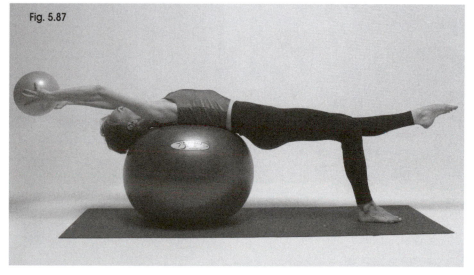

Fig. 5.87

2. Exhale to lift one foot and straighten the knee (fig. 5.86).
3. Hold steady for a couple of breaths.
4. Exhale to place the foot back on mat.
5. Inhale to prepare.
6. Exhale to lift the other foot and straighten the knee.
7. Hold steady for a couple of breaths.

8. Exhale to return. Repeat five times with each leg.
9. For an extra challenge write the alphabet with your foot when ready. Or take the small ball overhead and hold for a couple of breaths (fig. 5.87). Breathe naturally.

Body Openers

We spend too much time curling our bodies forward. Working on the ball opens your chest and lungs, stretches the spine and abdominals, and promotes relaxation. Exercising with the small ball gives you a stretch in the upper back, not just the flexible low back. Take your time in Body Openers; feel the length from the toes up to the crown of the head. To come out of these stretches place your hands behind your head and lift the head first. Then roll into a ball on your side, pulling your knees to your chest.

Purpose To stretch the spine, abdominals, and back of the neck.

Watchpoints • Make sure the neck is safe. Use a cushion under the head if necessary. • Be sure that long hair does not get stuck under the ball.

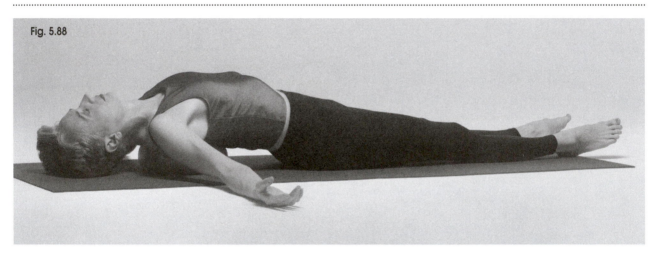

Fig. 5.88

starting position

Lie on your back. Roll to one side and slip the small ball between your shoulder blades or at the bottom of your shoulder blades and roll back onto the ball.

movement 1: upper chest opener

1. Clasp your hands behind your head and slowly lower the head, arching back over the ball. If desired, release the hands once the head is safely supported on the mat. Keep knees bent or straighten the legs down the mat (fig. 5.88).
2. Slowly circle the arms or simply rest here, taking a few deep breaths.

movement 2: upper chest opener with twist

1. Keep the knees bent. Clasp your hands behind your head and keep the head comfortable (fig. 5.89). Inhale.
2. Exhale and drop the knees to the right side while rotating the body to the left side. Feet stay on the mat. Keep the head supported by the hands (fig. 5.90).
3. Breathe in and out and repeat the twisting movement on the other side (fig. 5.91).
4. To come out of these stretches, place the hands behind the head and lift the head. Then roll into a ball on your side.

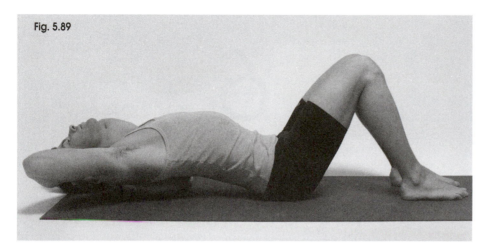

Fig. 5.89

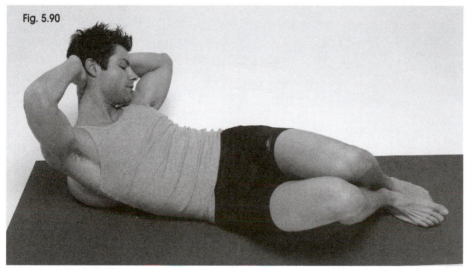

Fig. 5.90

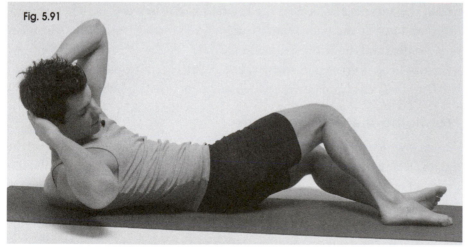

Fig. 5.91

6
Advanced Abs on the Ball

These are the most challenging exercises short of standing on a ball. By the time you reach the advanced level healthy movement patterns should ideally be in place, and the deep muscles should be functioning by themselves without your having to think about them. It is still a good idea to review the fundamentals at the beginning of all three sections. Warm up by using the Fifteen-minute Basic Abs Workout shown on page 162, and then cautiously add one or two advanced exercises at a time. After you have warmed up plan to add the advanced work near the beginning of your workout, when you are fresh, and not at the end. Watch fatigue levels—when fatigue sets in technique suffers and the wrong muscles take over.

Work in an open area in case you lose balance. Always use a burst-resistant ball: they will slowly deflate if accidentally punctured and will not explode.

Practicing the Fundamentals

As you practice the fundamentals in preparation for the advanced Abs on the Ball exercises, think quality not quantity. By now you realize how this abdominal workout differs from others. The emphasis as you move into the final two fundamentals is not how high you can lift a leg or an arm but whether you are able to maintain a precise contraction of the inner core, keeping neutral spine and optimal posture as you add the movement of the limbs.

Fundamental #1: One Leg Standing

It will be the strength of your core that will keep you from toppling over when balancing on one leg or arm. Draw your navel toward your spine and feel the crown of the head stretch upward as the foot grounds with the floor. Try these moves each day and hold them a bit longer each time. Close the eyes for extra challenge.

Purpose To tone the deep core muscles and challenge balance.

Watchpoints • Do not rush in or out of the balances. • Keep the shoulders relaxed. • Keep the pelvis in neutral, tailbone down.

starting position

Stand with both feet firmly planted on the ground. Fan out the toes and make sure the weight is evenly distributed on both feet and across both feet. Hold the large or small ball.

movement 1: the kite

1. Lift the ball overhead. Ground your right foot into the mat and shift the weight to that foot. Holding the ball in your hands, stretch the ball to the right side and move the left leg to the left, reaching it away from the body (fig. 6.1).
2. Take a few breaths, keeping the core strong. Find your center. Hold for 10 seconds.
3. Return so both feet are back on the mat. Repeat on the other side.

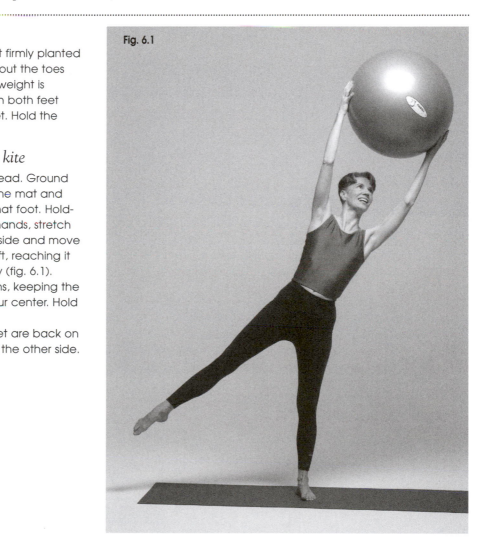

Fig. 6.1

117

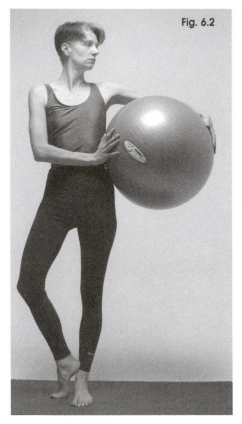

Fig. 6.2

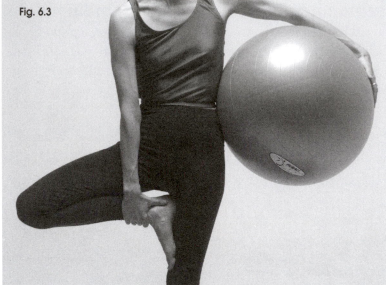

Fig. 6.3

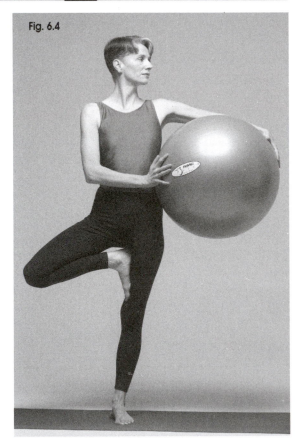

Fig. 6.4

movement 2: the tree

1. Ground your left foot into the mat and shift the weight to that foot as you hold the ball on the left side of the body. Lift the right foot to the ankle to begin (fig. 6.2).
2. When you have found your balance, take the right ankle with the right hand and lift the leg to the top of the inner thigh. If desired, place your foot lower on the leg but do not press the foot on the inside of the knee. Press the foot into the thigh, keeping the knee open (fig. 6.3).
3. Focus on a nonmoving point in front of you and hold for 20 to 30 seconds.
4. To further challenge your balance, turn the head to the side and hold (fig. 6.4).
5. Breathe smoothly. Repeat on the other side.

Fundamental #2: Opposite Hand and Foot

The upper and lower body work together in this exercise. Imagine that the navel is a mattress button. A thick cord connects the navel button to the spine. Gently pull on that cord, drawing the navel and the area between the navel and pubic bone away from the edge of your pants. Keep the navel-to-spine connection as you add the movement of the limbs. It is not important how high you lift the hand or foot but that you are able to maintain neutral spine as you extend the opposite hand and foot.

Purpose To tone the inner core, back, and buttocks muscles.

Watchpoints • The contraction of the abdominals is performed in a slow, controlled manner. Avoid arching the back or twisting the pelvis. Keep the hips on the ball and do not twist the hip up as you lift the leg. • Keep shoulders easing down the back and avoid letting the leg or arm rise above the height of the torso.

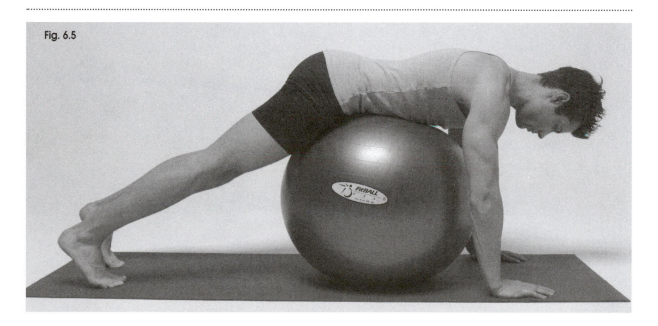

Fig. 6.5

starting position

Lie with the belly on the ball. Place the hands on the floor below the shoulders. Stretch the legs behind you, shoulder-distance apart (fig. 6.5).

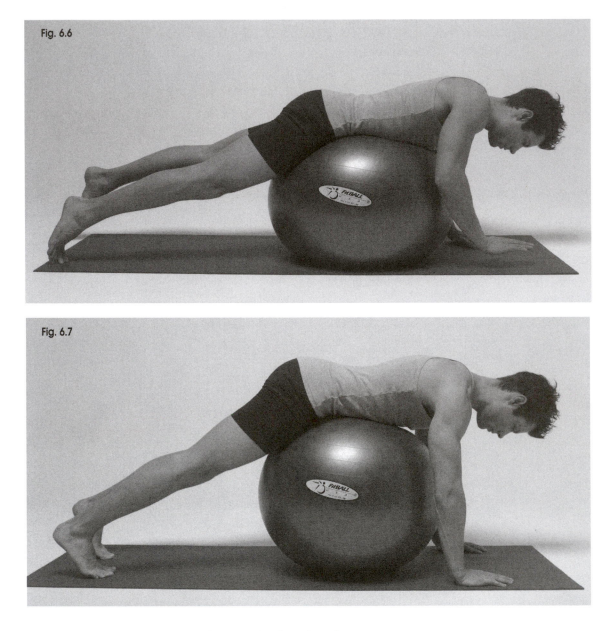

Fig. 6.6

Fig. 6.7

movement 1: opposite hand and foot, two inches

1. Inhale to lengthen through the spine.

2. Exhale to pull the navel toward the spine and simultaneously raise the right hand and left foot two inches off the mat (fig. 6.6).

3. Inhale to maintain the contraction and lower the hand and foot.

4. Exhale, keeping the navel in, and raise the left hand and right foot two inches off the mat.

5. Repeat four to six times on each side, keeping the abdominals connected for both the in and the out breaths.

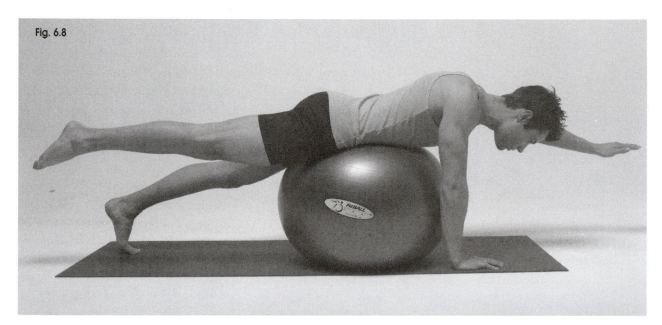

Fig. 6.8

movement 2: opposite hand and foot, full height

1. Inhale to lengthen through the spine (fig. 6.7).
2. Exhale to pull the navel in and simultaneously raise the right heel to buttocks height or lower and the left hand to shoulder height or lower. Hold for 5 to 20 seconds, breathing naturally (fig. 6.8).
3. Inhale to keep the contraction and lower the leg and hand.
4. Exhale to raise the left heel and right hand. Hold for 5 to 20 seconds, breathing naturally.
5. Repeat four to six times on each side, keeping the abdominals connected for both the in and the out breaths.

The Advanced Abs on the Ball Exercises

Remember, it is not merely the strength of the outer layer that allows you to perform these challenging moves. The strength of the deep inner core is key. The more efficiently the deep stabilizing muscles work to support the pelvis and low back against the movements of the limbs, the more you will be able to swing, throw, kick, or absorb forces in your sport or recreational activities. In addition, if you are working the core properly you should feel less tension in the jaw, neck, shoulders, wrists, and low back. If the core is not properly supporting the forces of the legs and arms, the body will compensate by using the wrong muscles and moving into positions that are not optimal.

The Hundred

This invigorating exercise gets the blood circulating and warms the body as you coordinate movement with breathing. Pump the arms up and down as if on a bed of springs as you inhale for five counts and exhale for five counts. Do not lift higher than the base of the shoulder blades. Squeeze the small ball as you lower the legs to a 45-degree angle (or lower) on the exhalation. Lift the legs on the inhale. Use the exhalation to scoop the navel and keep the low back on the mat as you lower the legs.

Purpose To challenge the abdominals and warm up the body.

Watchpoints • Make sure the entire arm moves from the socket. Do not move from the wrist or the elbow. • Keep the elbows soft, not hyperextended. • Do not let the torso move with the pumps. • Keep the shoulders down.

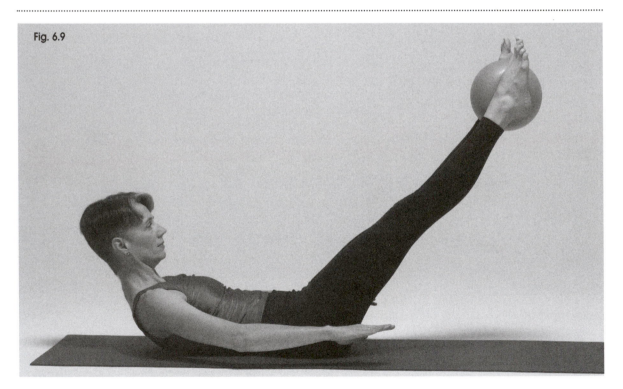

Fig. 6.9

starting position

Lie on your back and bring your knees to your chest. Place the small ball between your ankles.

movement: the hundred

1. Inhale to prepare. Exhale to curl up, extending your legs and stretching your arms past your thighs. Your gaze is on your knees, not on the ceiling (fig. 6.9).

2. Inhale and exhale for five breaths, squeezing the ball on each exhalation. With each breath pump your arms as if they are on a bed of springs. Elbows are soft.

3. Maintain this position, breathing for 100 counts.

4. Finish by bending the knees to the chest and lowering the head to the mat.

Roll Over

This exercise is difficult to teach in a group class because most students, even advanced students, do not have the strength or ability to organize the entire body so as not to put pressure on the neck. Placing the small ball under the hips is an excellent way to approach this highly controlled movement. Think of peeling away from the mat one vertebra at a time, using the abdominals, not the arms, to lift the legs overhead. Do not take your weight so far back that you are crunching onto the neck. Keep your head aligned on your spine.

Purpose To strengthen lower and upper abdominals and improve flexibility in the low back and hamstrings.

Watchpoints • Avoid using the hands to help you get the legs overhead—use the abdominals. • Keep the navel-to-spine connection. • Keep your head aligned on the spine. • Avoid this exercise if you have neck or low-back problems.

....

starting position

Lie on your back and tuck the small ball under your hips. Bring the knees up to the chest and extend your legs to the ceiling at a 90-degree angle to the floor (fig. 6.10).

movement 1: small ball at ankles

1. Use a second ball at the ankles (or no ball); hold the ball at the hips in place with your hands. Inhale to prepare.

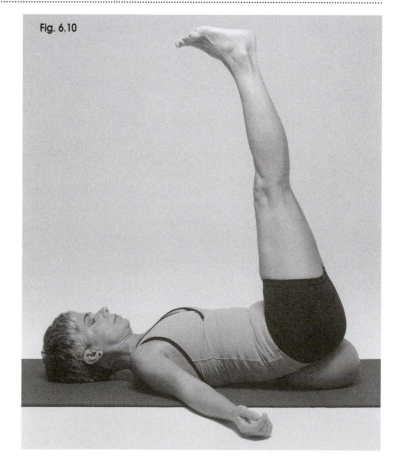
Fig. 6.10

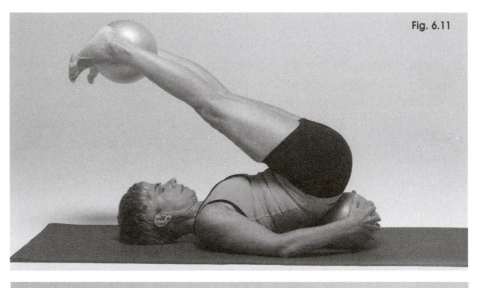

Fig. 6.11

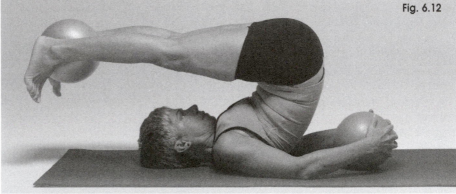

Fig. 6.12

2. Engaging your abdominals, exhale to peel away from the small ball and extend the legs overhead (fig. 6.11).

3. Stop when the legs are parallel to the floor. Inhale and gently squeeze the ball with your hands. Flex the feet if desired (fig. 6.12).

4. Exhale to roll down through the spine one vertebra at a time (fig. 6.13). Lower your feet to the starting position. Keep the low back from popping off the mat.

5. Repeat three to five times.

movement 2: large ball between ankles

1. Legs are extended to the ceiling at a 90-degree angle with the large ball between the feet (fig. 6.14). Inhale to prepare.

2. Using your abdominals, exhale to peel away from the mat and extend the legs overhead.

3. Stop when the legs are parallel to the floor. Inhale and gently squeeze the ball (fig. 6.15). Flex the feet if desired.

4. Exhale to roll down through the spine one vertebra at a time (fig. 6.16). Lower the ball to an angle at which you are able to keep your low back on the mat.

5. Repeat three to five times.

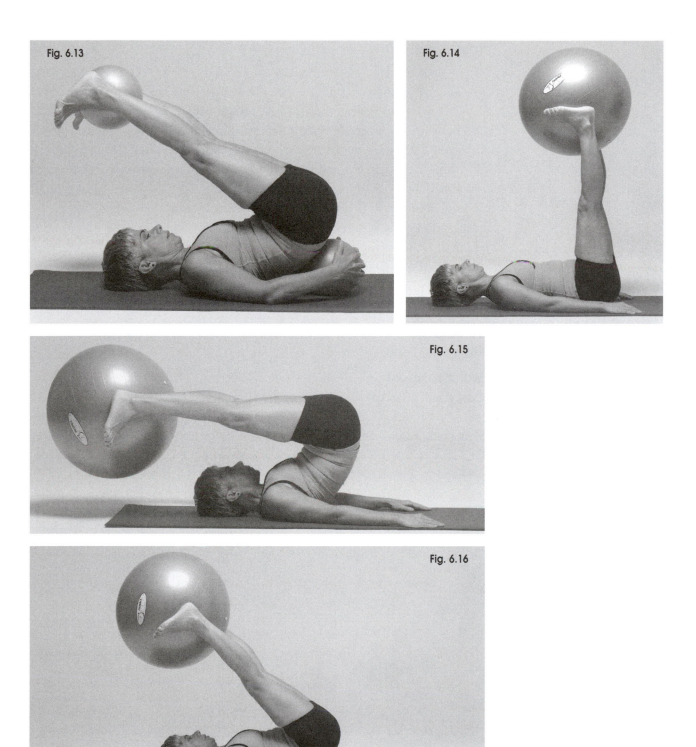

Fig. 6.13

Fig. 6.14

Fig. 6.15

Fig. 6.16

Corkscrew

The Corkscrew is in the same family as the Pilates Roll Over. Continue to use the deep abdominals to stabilize the pelvis against the movement of the heavy legs. Keep circles small to begin with and use your arms beside you for stability. Later try the exercise with the arms in a T-shape. Sweep the legs in one direction, accentuating the upswing, and alternate the direction of the circle. The hips remain on the mat or on the small ball in movements 1 and 2. The small ball under the hips will help those with a tight low back. Movement 3 is similar to the Roll Over, except you are rolling down on one side of the spine and rolling up on the other. Keep your arms close to the body—press them into the mat and anchor the body with them as you lift the legs and take them overhead. Once the legs are overhead, shift the weight over to one side of the spine and then slowly roll down through the spine. Remember to alternate the direction of the circle at the top of the movement.

Purpose Targets the low abdominals, hip flexors, trunk stability, and inner thighs and buttocks.

Watchpoints • In movements 1 and 2 keep hips on the mat or the ball and keep the low back stable. • As you are circling the legs low in the front do not allow your back to arch off the mat. • Try to keep tension out of the neck, shoulders, and jaw. • Avoid if you have neck or low-back problems.

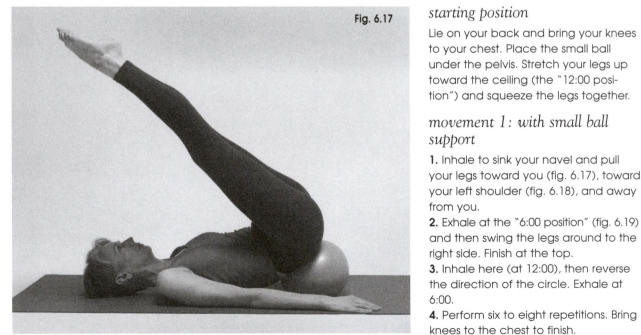

Fig. 6.17

starting position

Lie on your back and bring your knees to your chest. Place the small ball under the pelvis. Stretch your legs up toward the ceiling (the "12:00 position") and squeeze the legs together.

movement 1: with small ball support

1. Inhale to sink your navel and pull your legs toward you (fig. 6.17), toward your left shoulder (fig. 6.18), and away from you.

2. Exhale at the "6:00 position" (fig. 6.19) and then swing the legs around to the right side. Finish at the top.

3. Inhale here (at 12:00), then reverse the direction of the circle. Exhale at 6:00.

4. Perform six to eight repetitions. Bring knees to the chest to finish.

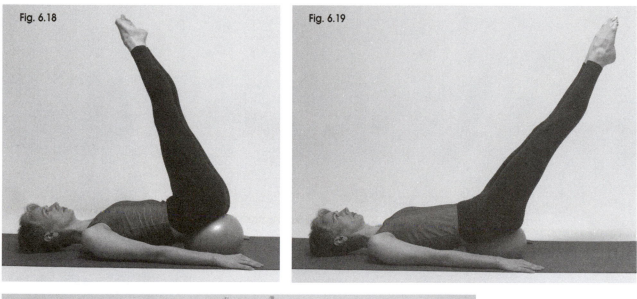

Fig. 6.18

Fig. 6.19

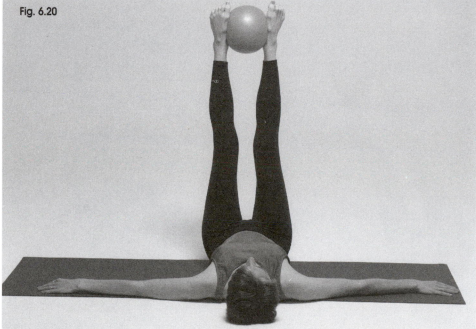

Fig. 6.20

movement 2: corkscrew prep

1. Take the small ball out from under the pelvis and place it between the ankles. Stretch the legs into the air. Arms can be beside you on the mat or stretched out in a T-shape (fig. 6.20).

2. Inhale to pull your navel in and circle your legs to the left (fig. 6.21), then away from you.

3. Exhale at 6:00, then sweep the legs to the other side (fig. 6.22), finishing at the top.

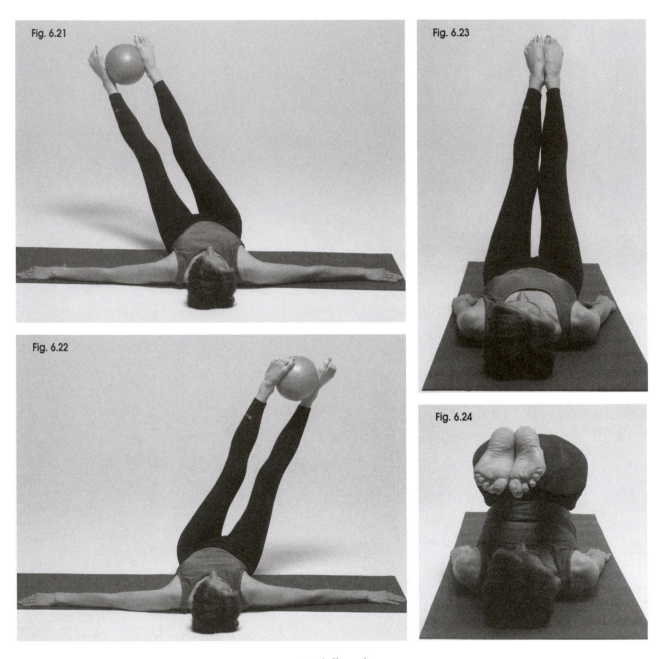

Fig. 6.21

Fig. 6.22

Fig. 6.23

Fig. 6.24

4. Inhale at 12:00, then reverse the direction of the circle. Exhale at 6:00.
5. Perform six to eight repetitions. Bring knees to the chest to finish.

movement 3: full corkscrew

1. Put the small ball to the side and stretch the legs into the air. Stretch your arms alongside your body and press them into the mat (fig. 6.23).
2. Inhale to prepare.

3. Initiating with your abdominals, on the exhale take the legs straight overhead so that the legs are parallel to the floor (fig. 6.24).
4. Inhale and shift your hips slightly to the right side (fig. 6.25). Roll down

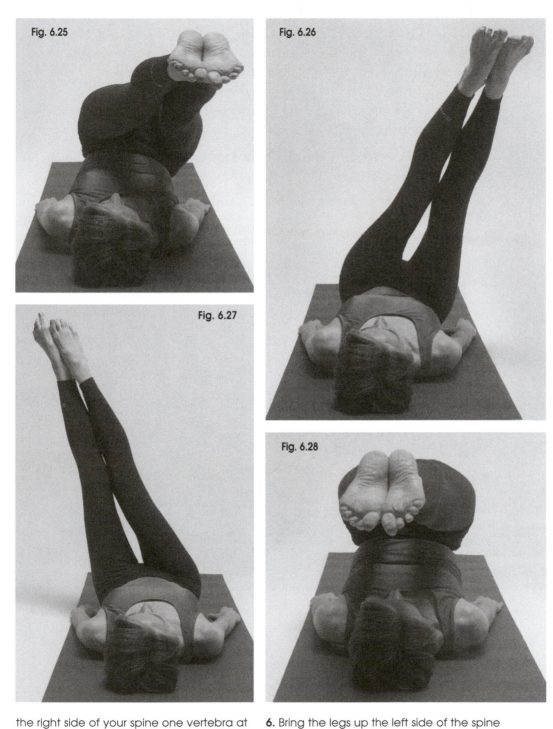

Fig. 6.25

Fig. 6.26

Fig. 6.27

Fig. 6.28

the right side of your spine one vertebra at a time (fig. 6.26).

5. At 6:00, taking care to keep the low back on the mat, exhale and circle the legs around to the left side (fig. 6.27).

6. Bring the legs up the left side of the spine and back overhead to center (fig. 6.28).

7. Alternate the direction of the circle. Perform three repetitions in each direction.

Side Bridge on Small Ball

Side Bridge on a mobile surface makes the muscles on the side of the body work very hard. You might want to first try this exercise without a ball and on a stable surface. Keep the navel pulled in to engage the deep inner corset so as not to sink in the middle, and keep the body supported on the strong elbow. Do not sink the shoulder or elbow.

Purpose To strengthen the quadratus lumborum, abdominal obliques, and deep abdominals.

Watchpoints • Keep the spine straight, steady, and in neutral. • Keep one hip stacked on top of the other. Kneecaps and hips face forward. • Make sure to maintain the navel-to-spine connection.

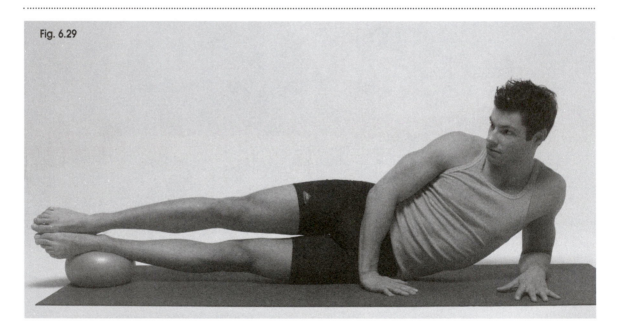

Fig. 6.29

starting position

Begin on your side supported by your hips and elbows. Place the free hand on the mat to help you get into position (fig. 6.29).

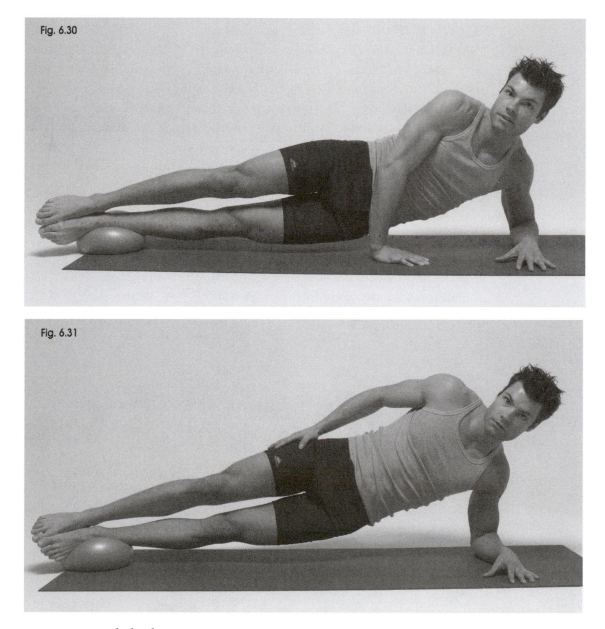

Fig. 6.30

Fig. 6.31

movement: side bridge

1. Place lower heel on the small ball. Stack the other heel on top and lift into a side plank position (fig. 6.30).
2. When you're steady, lift the hand that is on the mat and place it on your thigh (fig. 6.31). Breathe naturally and hold for 5 to 10 seconds.
3. Lower your body and repeat four times.
4. Move to the other side.

Boomerang

This Pilates Advanced Challenge combines the Roll Over and the Teaser. (See Roll Over on page 123 and Teaser on page 139.) It is not necessary to roll back on your neck, and the legs can be bent in the Teaser position to make the move more accessible. However, do this exercise very precisely and with a great deal of control to avoid sloppiness. There should be a continuous flow from one position to the next. The abdominal core will help you maintain your balance so that you do not simply drop the legs near the end of the move.

Purpose To strengthen many muscles in the body, especially the abdominal core and hip flexors. To practice coordination and balance.

Watchpoints • Avoid rolling back and placing weight onto the neck area; only go as far as the upper back. • Resist the urge to drop the legs quickly to the mat at the end of the exercise. Use the strength of the abdominals and the hip flexors to slowly lower the legs with control. • Avoid this exercise if you have shoulder or neck problems.

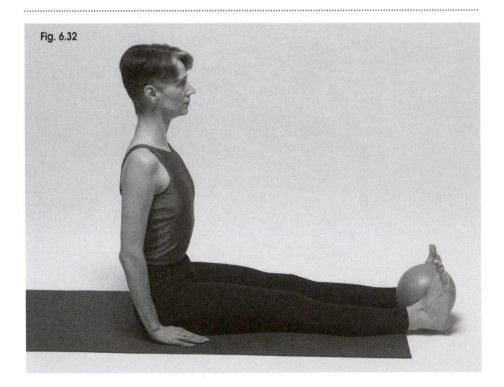

Fig. 6.32

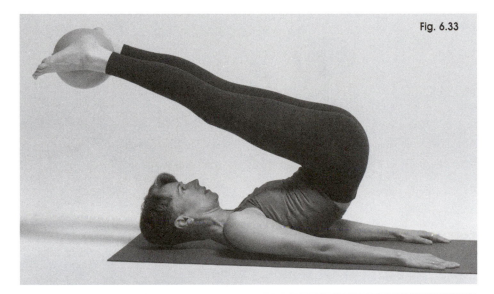

Fig. 6.33

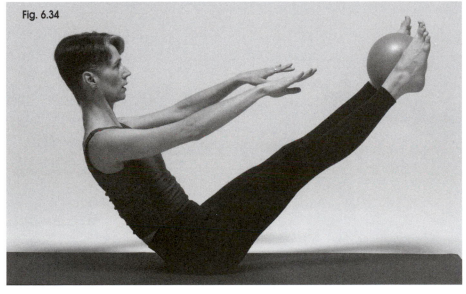

Fig. 6.34

starting position

Sit very tall on your sitz bones with the small ball between your ankles. Place the hands on the mat directly below your shoulders (fig. 6.32).

movement: the boomerang

1. Inhale to grow tall.

2. Exhale to sink the navel and roll back, lifting your legs off the mat. Take the legs overhead without using the arms to aid you (fig. 6.33).
3. Inhale to gently squeeze the ball.
4. Exhale to smoothly roll back and up to the Teaser position, stretching your hands toward the toes (fig. 6.34).
5. Keeping the body balanced here,

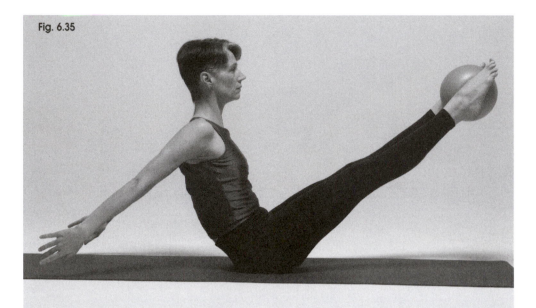

Fig. 6.35

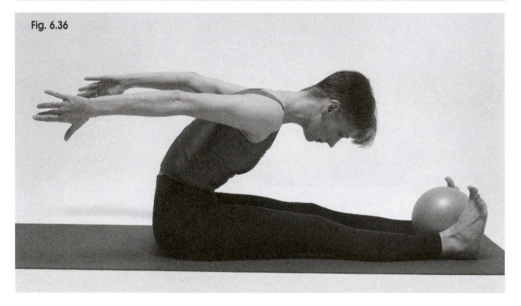

Fig. 6.36

inhale to sweep the fingertips in a wide circle around to the back (fig. 6.35). Sustain this position.

6. Exhale to *slowly* lower the legs to the mat as the arms stretch back. Use the reaching back of the arms to counterbalance the weight of the heavy legs. As your legs arrive on the mat curl the upper body over the legs. Keep the navel lifted (fig. 6.36).

7. Inhale to circle your arms forward, as wide and as high as possible, toward your toes. Lengthen through the neck and keep shoulders stabilized and not lifted to your ears.

8. Exhale to roll up tall to the starting position.

9. Repeat four to six times.

Rocking Horse Extension

Rocking Horse is an excellent way to train the core and to coordinate the upper body with the lower body. Keep the body very stable. When you lower the upper body the legs will lift and make a long bow shape as they come up slightly into the air. As the legs lower the upper body will lift. A very soggy small ball on the pelvis makes the pubic bone comfortable. As you rock forward control the motion with your hands and keep the elbows in tight to the body. Keep the legs very straight.

Purpose To stretch and strengthen the abdominals and work the spinal muscles, gluteals, and the back of legs.

Watchpoints • Keep length in the back of the neck and spine. • Keep the navel-to-spine connection. • Keep the shoulders sliding down the back.

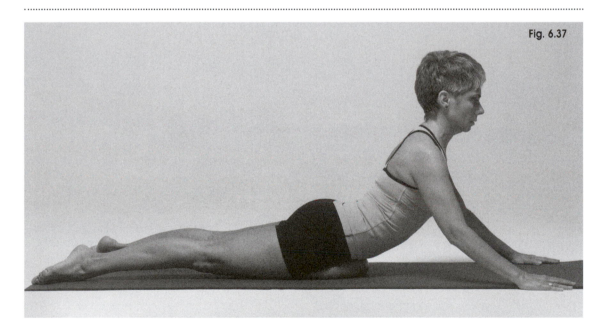

Fig. 6.37

starting position

Lie on your belly and place a very soggy ball under the pelvis. The small ball should only be inflated to half of its capacity (see the ball in fig. 6.39 on page 136). Place your hands just in front of your shoulders, palms down. Elbows are close to the body and point toward the feet. Gaze at the mat. Add a small ball between the ankles for extra challenge.

movement: rocking horse

1. Inhale to slide the shoulder blades downward.
2. Exhale to lift the navel and the breastbone, extending the spine. Your neck is long. Your gaze is straight ahead (fig. 6.37).

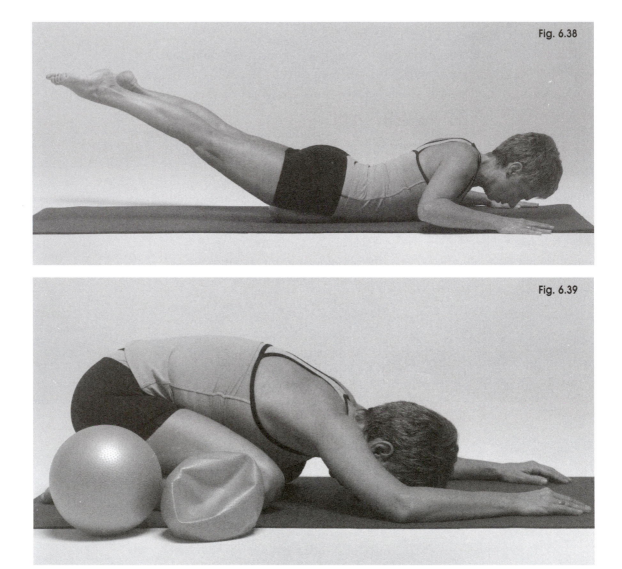

Fig. 6.38

Fig. 6.39

3. Inhale to connect through the gluteals and the hamstrings. Stretch the legs up and away from you.
4. Exhale to rock forward, lifting the legs in the air (fig. 6.38). Keep the legs very straight. Keep the elbows close to the

body and the head aligned on spine.
5. Inhale to rock the body back up.
6. Repeat three to five times.
7. Afterward stretch out the back in Shell (fig. 6.39).

Scissors

Keep the core very stable and strong as you add a scissor action of the legs. Pulse the lifted leg twice, tapping the front of the ankle or shin against the ball each time. Take care that the elbows are soft and not locked. Keep the shoulders sliding down the back. If you have neck strain put your head on the mat while doing the exercise. If you have a tight low back or hamstrings, start by bending the legs.

Purpose To strengthen legs and abdominals.

Watchpoints • Keep the shoulders from lifting as you take the ball overhead.
• Keep the navel pulled in and make sure the abdominals are not popping out.

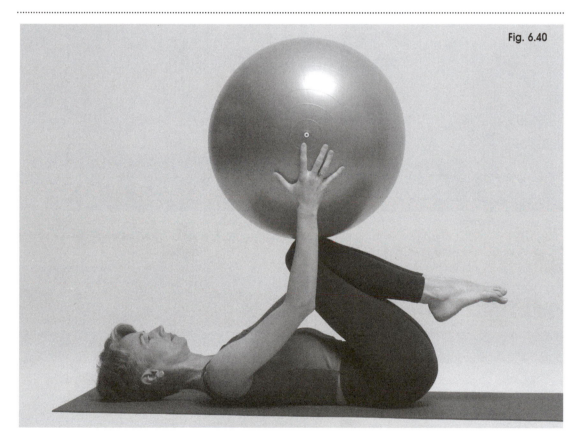

Fig. 6.40

starting position

Lie on the mat. Bring the knees up to the chest. Hold the ball with both hands and place the ball on the shins (fig. 6.40).

movement: scissors

1. Inhale to curl the head and upper body, holding the ball on the shins.

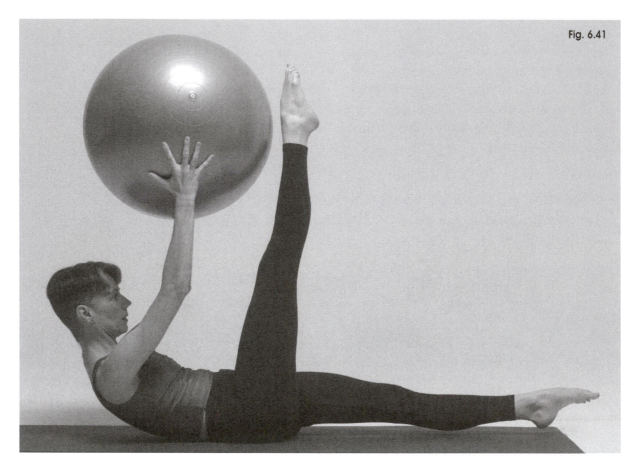

Fig. 6.41

2. Exhale to split the legs and tap the right leg twice against the ball (fig. 6.41).
3. Inhale to switch legs.
4. Exhale to split the legs and tap the left leg twice against the ball.

5. Repeat six to eight times, keeping the legs straight.
6. Finish by curling the body, knees to the chest and head on the mat.

Ball-in-the-Hands Challenge

*b*e aware of how the large ball held between the hands may change your shoulder position, head alignment, and elbow placement. One of the challenges of Abs on the Ball is trying not to allow the ball to distort the body or distract you from performing the exercise with precision.

Whenever the ball, large or small, is placed into the hands, the elbows must *always* be soft and not locked. The larger the ball the more unwieldy it is. In advanced exercises like Scissors and Teaser it may be better to master the move first with a small ball and only add the large ball when you are sure that it will not tempt the body back into faulty movement patterns or incorrect posture, or add strain.

The ball is a partner in your mat work, not just a prop. Practice and a strong mind-body connection will ensure that the ball is handled with fluidity and control.

Teaser

The Pilates Teaser is not only an intense test for your abdominals, but it increases balance and control as you roll the body up and down. Make sure you are ready for this exercise. If you have a sensitive low back, bend the knees. Take care that the large ball does not allow you to lift your shoulders up to your ears. The ball should help float you up, not weigh you down.

Purpose To strengthen the abdominals and practice articulating through the spine.

Watchpoints • Neck and shoulders should be relaxed. • Lift from the chest and not the head as you peel off the mat and into the air. Use the exhalation to help you up.

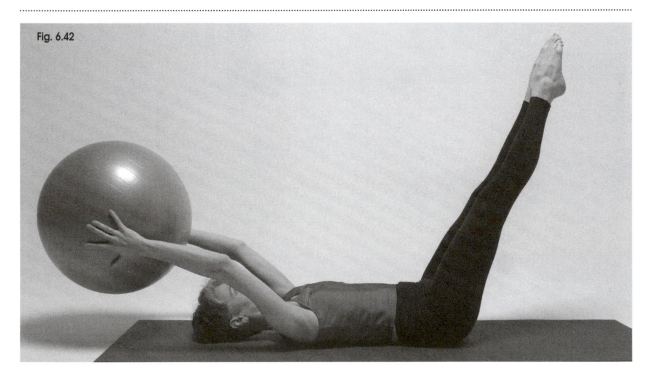

Fig. 6.42

starting position

Lie on your back. Extend the legs into the air and turn them out from the hip sockets. Squeeze the inner thighs and buttocks. Take the large ball overhead (fig. 6.42).

movement 1: straight legs in air

1. Inhale to bring the ball to the ceiling. On the exhalation press your sacrum into the mat and continue the movement forward so that your head and upper body follow the ball. You will be balancing just back of your sitz bones.

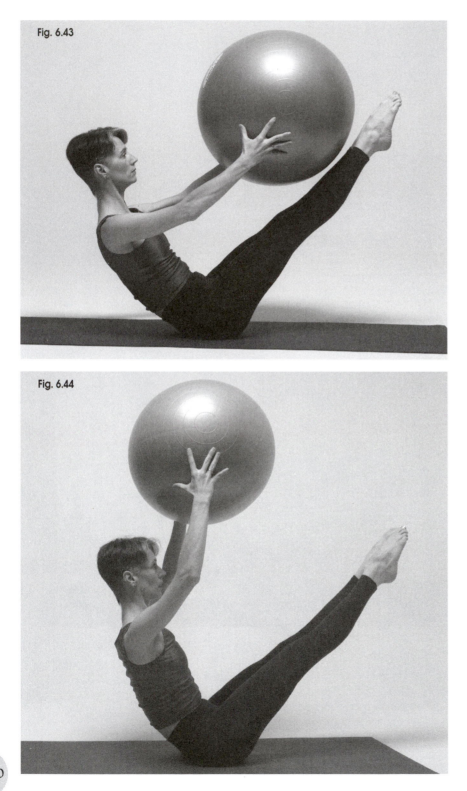

Fig. 6.43

Fig. 6.44

Arms will be parallel to legs. Scoop the belly and hold (fig. 6.43).

2. Inhale to lift the ball back slightly so that the arms are just in front of the ears but the shoulders remain down (fig. 6.44).

3. Exhale to drop the navel and roll your spine back down, pressing one bone at a time into the mat.

4. Return to the starting position with the ball overhead.

5. Repeat six times.

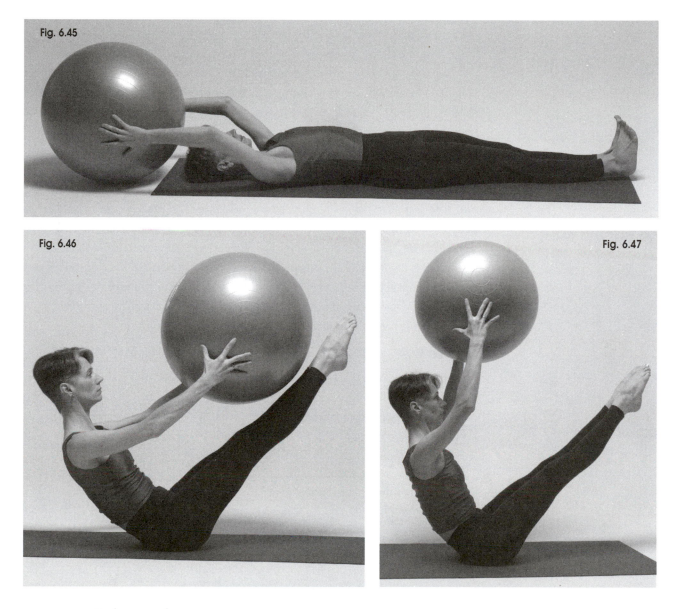

Fig. 6.45

Fig. 6.46

Fig. 6.47

movement 2: legs on the mat

1. Lie flat on your back with legs long. Holding the ball, reach your arms back overhead. Keep the abdominal connection to ensure that your rib cage is not popping out (fig. 6.45).

2. On the exhale press your sacrum into the mat and stretch your arms and lift your legs simultaneously. Balance as close to your sitz bones as possible.

Scoop the belly and hold (fig. 6.46).

3. Inhale to lift the ball back slightly so that the arms come to the ears or slightly in front, but the shoulders remain down (fig. 6.47).

4. Exhale to drop the navel and roll your spine back down, pressing one bone at a time into the mat. Simultaneously roll through the spine and lower the legs.

5. Repeat six times.

Sidebend and Twist

This very challenging exercise is taken from the Pilates mat repertoire. Adding the ball to the exercise supports the body so that some of the body's weight is taken off the wrist, but good shoulder strength and shoulder stabilization are still needed. Avoid this exercise if you have wrist, shoulder, or neck problems. The ball makes movement 2, the Twist, more accessible for most people. Master the Sidebend first. This is not just a side stretch. Think of it more as a side plank: you need to place the hip on the center top of the ball and get the body weight up and over the ball. Weight should go onto the arm that is placed directly below the shoulder on the mat. There should be at least two inches between the ball and the supporting arm. Do not sink into the ball; use it merely as a support. When you go into the Twist use the abdominals to pike the hips upward, as if you are suspended from above. Keep the supporting shoulder strong and stable by recruiting the muscles under the armpit and across the side of the chest. In the top position there should be a long line from the shoulders through the hip, knees, and toes.

Purpose Works abdominals, obliques, back, and upper body.

Watchpoints • In the side plank or Sidebend positions, make sure the hand is directly below the shoulder and that you are recruiting the muscles under the armpit. • Try to lift out of your shoulder, one hip on top of the other. • Don't let the shoulders lift up to your ears. • Avoid this exercise if you have wrist or shoulder problems.

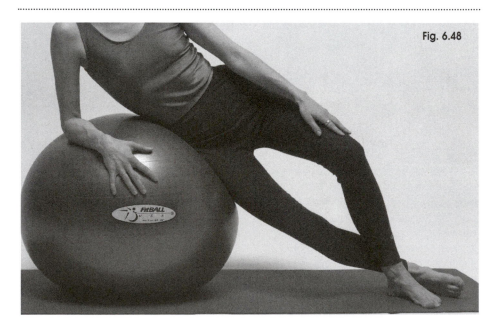

Fig. 6.48

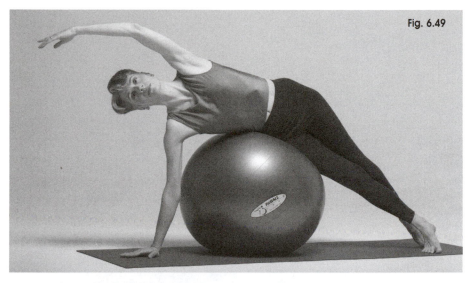

Fig. 6.49

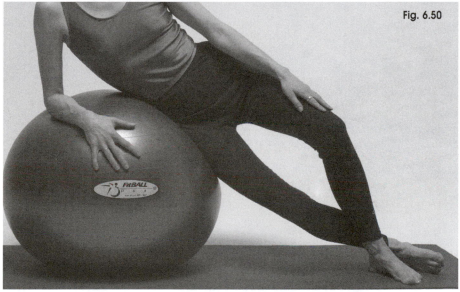

Fig. 6.50

starting position

Cross your left foot in front of your right leg and begin by placing the side of the hip on the top center of the ball. Shift your weight onto the ball. Your left arm rests on the left thigh (fig. 6.48).

movement 1: sidebend

1. Inhale to prepare. Exhale to lift the hips toward the ceiling as you stretch the body across the ball, placing the hand two inches or more away from the ball. The palm of your hand should be on the mat directly under your shoulders. Come into a side plank, lifting your hips and stretching your arm overhead close to your ear. Maintain one hip on top of the other (fig. 6.49).

2. Inhale to bend the knees slightly and rest the hips on the ball. Return to starting position, lowering the left arm to rest on the thigh (fig. 6.50).

3. Repeat three times and change sides.

143

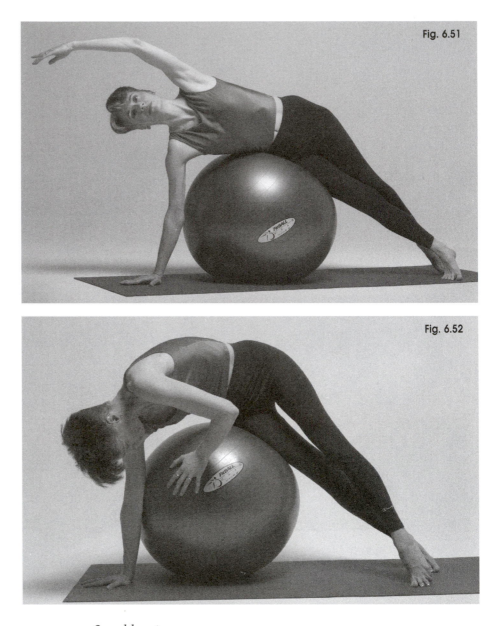

Fig. 6.51

Fig. 6.52

movement 2: add twist

1. Take the same starting position as Sidebend. Come into a side plank, lifting your hips and stretching your left arm overhead close to your ear. The right hand should be on the mat directly under your shoulder (fig. 6.51).

2. Inhale to sweep the left arm to touch the ball (fig. 6.52). Continuing the motion, exhale to pull up the navel and pike the hips toward the ceiling, straightening the legs and rotating the torso toward the mat. Stretch the crown of the head away from your hips and roll the ball behind you. Keep your

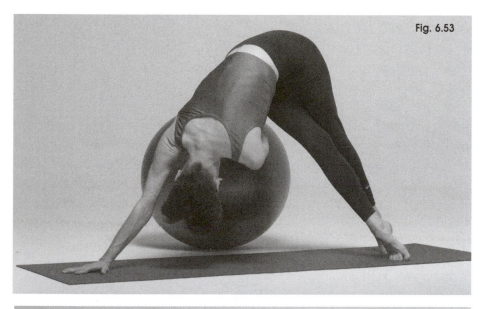

Fig. 6.53

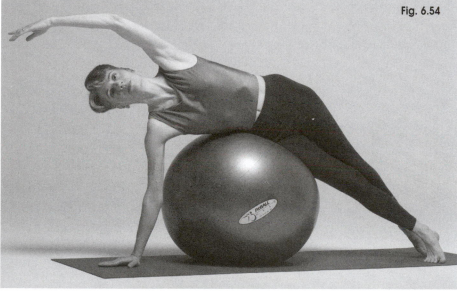

Fig. 6.54

hand on the ball and follow it with your
eyes (fig. 6.53).
3. Inhale to return the ball to your hip.
4. Exhale to swivel back and return to

the side plank, lifting your hips and
stretching your arm overhead close to
your ear (fig. 6.54).
5. Repeat twice and change sides.

Side-twist Plank

This exercise is usually easier on one side, as one oblique muscle group is often stronger than the other. What is important is to keep shoulders and head completely oriented down toward the mat, as you do in the ordinary Plank position. The upper body does not change; you simply swivel your body as one unit and line up your hipbones one on top of the other, perpendicular to the floor. Notice that one elbow will bend more than the other. The abdominals must be engaged to protect the low back and prevent the body from sagging in the middle. Keep your body "stiff as a board," and the legs must stay straight. Again, the most difficult part of this exercise comes after you have worked both sides: it will feel like a long walk back until you are safely on the mat.

Purpose To work the abdominals, obliques, and upper body.

Watchpoints • Maintain good stability in the shoulder girdle. • Keep your shoulder blades open across the back and down, not up by the ears. Elbows are slightly soft and angling back at a 45-degree angle. • Do not let the head drop; keep it in line with the spine. • Keep the legs glued together so that one does not move forward of the other.

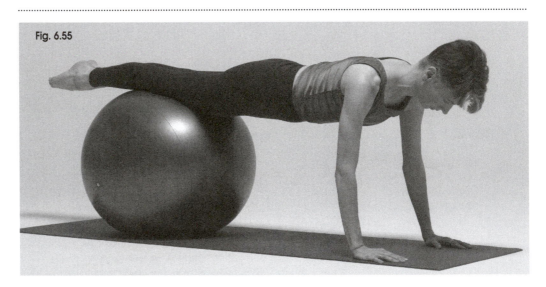

Fig. 6.55

starting position

Kneel in front of the ball. Place hands palm down on the floor.

movement: side-twist plank

1. Walk out until the ball is on the thighs. For more challenge walk out

until the ball is on the shins, keeping hands just wider than the shoulders. Fingertips should be parallel to the body, elbows angled slightly back. Do not let the midline drop. Keep legs very straight and turned out, with the buttocks working and the navel lifted (fig. 6.55).

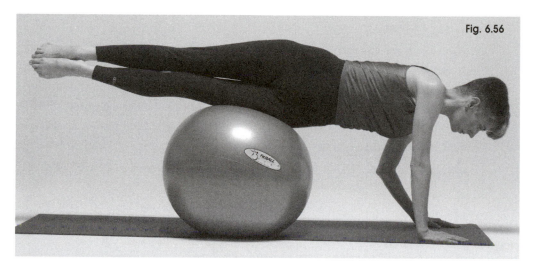

Fig. 6.56

2. Hold for a second and breathe naturally.
3. Keeping your head and shoulders exactly where they are, swivel the lower body until you lift one hip and place it directly on top of the other. Legs are straight. Gaze stays on the mat (fig. 6.56).

4. Hold for a number of seconds, breathing naturally.
5. Return to front Plank position.
6. Swivel to the other side and hold for a number of seconds.
7. Return by swiveling back into Plank and walking the hands back toward the ball. Repeat three times.

Abs on the Ball Fundamentals—A Review

- The deepest and most important abdominal muscle, the transversus abdominis, supports the spine by narrowing the abdominal wall. To locate the transversus place the tips of your three longest fingers one inch in from your hip bones and cough. With the correct contraction you will feel a tension in your fingertips as the abdominal wall narrows.

- Inhale through the nose, exhale through the mouth. On the exhalation make sure the navel is gently pulled in and the abdominals are activated. Think of sending the breath into the back of the rib cage, not the belly.

- Each exercise is initiated by gently drawing in between navel and pubic bone to activate the deep abdominal muscles and protect the spine.

- Watch that the abdominals do not bulge out, a sure sign the deep connection has been lost.

- Pelvic floor muscles connect through the nervous system to the deep abdominals. Engaging the pelvic floor "elevator" will help locate the deep abdominal connection.

- Neutral pelvis places the pelvis in the safest position and facilitates the best contraction of the deep abdominals. When lying on your back in neutral pelvis, the two hip bones on the front of the pelvis and the pubic bone are on the same plane. There is a small natural curve in the low back.

- Stabilize the powerhouse to prevent injuries in work, sports, and everyday life. Abdominal and low-back strength and endurance can heal and prevent low-back pain and poor posture.

The Pike

The Pike is an advanced move intended to challenge an already strong body. Imagine that you are suspended from the abdominals by a strong spring attached to the ceiling. Try to keep the legs absolutely straight and connected as you attempt to lift the pelvis with the abdominals. Once you are securely in the Pike, drop the head and look at the ball. Be sure the area around you is clear in case you lose your balance.

Purpose To strengthen abdominals, arms, and back. This exercise teaches balance.

Watchpoints • The body and legs must be rigid as a board. • Keep the torso steady while in the Pike, shoulders down and in place.

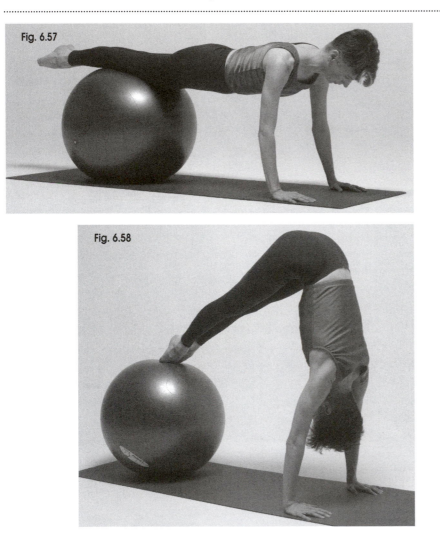

Fig. 6.57

Fig. 6.58

starting position

Kneel in front of the ball. Place your hands palm down on the floor. Walk out until the ball is on the shins or ankles. Hands are on the mat shoulder-distance apart or wider. Fingertips are parallel to the body.

movement 1: the pike

1. Be sure that the entire torso is in place: buttocks and inner thighs connected, head aligned on spine and not dropped (fig. 6.57). Inhale to prepare.

2. Using your abdominals, exhale to lift the pelvis as high as possible. Do not let the legs bend. The head will drop to remain aligned with the spine (fig. 6.58).

3. Inhale to lower to the Plank position.

4. Exhale to lift into the Pike. Go as high as you can without losing control.

5. Hold for a few counts, breathing naturally.

6. Repeat four to six times.

7. Return to Plank position and walk the hands back toward the ball.

Single Leg Shell

Alternate these advanced moves so that you are not doing Sidebends, Side-twist Plank, Pike, and Single Leg Shell all on the same day. It is essential for Single Leg Shell that the ball is in the correct place. It cannot be on the pelvis; it must be on the bottom of the thighs, near the knee but not putting any pressure on the knee. Activate the low abdominals and the hip muscles to draw the ball in toward your body and away. Control the ball—do not let the ball control you.

Purpose To strengthen the core. To practice balance and coordination.

Watchpoints • Make sure the ball is directly in front of the knees each time (Plank position) or you will not be in the right position when you roll up into Shell. • Do not sag in the midriff when you return to Plank position.

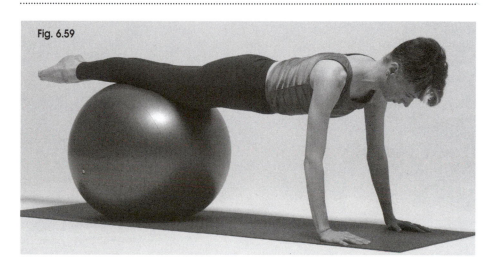

Fig. 6.59

starting position

Kneel in front of your ball. Crawl over the ball and walk out so that the hands are directly below the shoulders and the ball is directly in front of the knees, on the thighs. Squeeze thighs together and keep the sides of the knees touching each other (fig. 6.59).

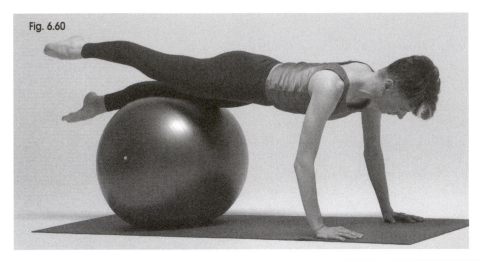

Fig. 6.60

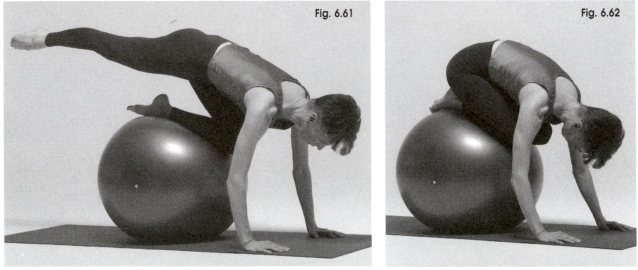

Fig. 6.61

Fig. 6.62

movement: single leg shell

1. Inhale to lengthen through the spine in Plank position. Lift the right leg off the ball (fig. 6.60).

2. Exhale to use the abdominals and the left knee to pull the ball under you. Leave the hands firmly planted where they are on the mat (fig. 6.61).

3. Inhale to bring the right knee in to meet the left knee (fig. 6.62). You should be in Shell position on the ball.

4. Exhale to use both legs to take the ball straight back to Plank position.

5. Repeat three or four times, alternating legs.

6. Finish in Plank position. Then pick up the hands and walk them toward the ball.

Kneeling Side Lifts

In this exercise the torso should remain very still while the leg moves. Keep the leg straight and image that you are circling the leg from the hip socket, not from the ankle or the knee. The kneecap should remain forward.

Purpose To strengthen the core and practice balance and coordination. To work the hips, buttocks, and thighs.

Watchpoints • Do not sink the shoulders or the waist as you lift the leg. • Avoid this exercise if you have bad knees. • Keep the elevated leg in line with the body. Only lift as high as you can manage to keep the torso steady.

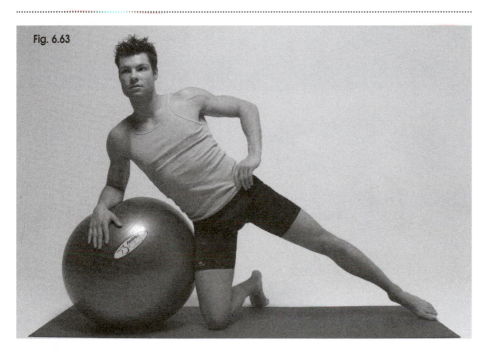

Fig. 6.63

starting position

Kneel beside your ball. Place your forearm on the ball and straighten your leg beside you. Place your hand on your hip. Stand upright on the knee closest to the ball (fig. 6.63). Keep your head aligned in the middle of your shoulders.

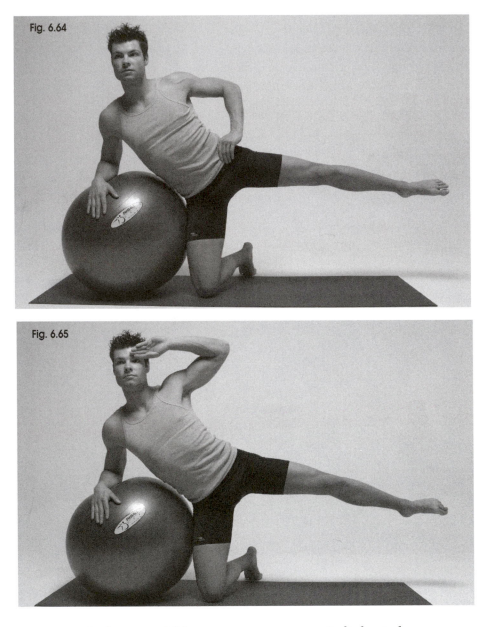

Fig. 6.64

Fig. 6.65

movement 1: lower and lift

1. Inhale to tighten your abdominals and stretch the leg away from you to lift it to hip height (fig. 6.64).
2. Exhale to press the leg down, resisting gravity.
3. Inhale to lift. Exhale to press down.
4. Repeat eight times.

movement 2: little circles

1. Inhale to tighten your abdominals and stretch the leg away from you to lift it to hip height. Place your hand on your forehead.
2. Breathing naturally, make five small circles forward and then five circles in reverse (fig. 6.65). Keep your torso steady.
3. Repeat on the other side.

The Star

We start this tricky balance posture by making sure the feet are in the proper place. Turn the foot so that the entire side surface is dug into the mat. Then stack one foot on top of the other and only lift the leg after you have found your balance. When you lift the leg try to keep the hips squared to the front and the foot flexed. Use the ball to support you but do not sink into the ball.

Purpose To strengthen the core and practice balance.

Watchpoints • Keep your core very stable and straight; your body should be like a board. • Do not allow your shoulders to lift.

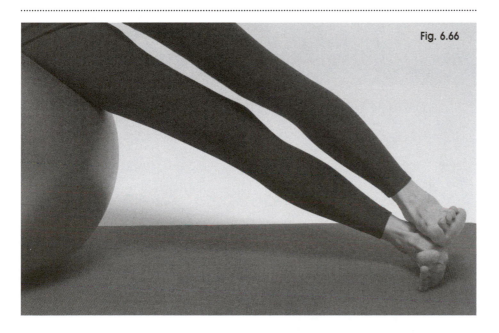

Fig. 6.66

starting position

Kneel beside the ball and climb sideways onto it, making sure the hip—not the rib cage—is on the ball. Open your legs shoulder-distance apart to begin; the top leg is in front. Support one arm on the ball.

movement: the star

1. Find your balance and narrow your base of support so that the side of one foot is digging into the mat and the other foot is stacked on top (fig. 6.66). Inhale to prepare.
2. Exhale to straighten the body into a side plank. Do not sink into the ball or

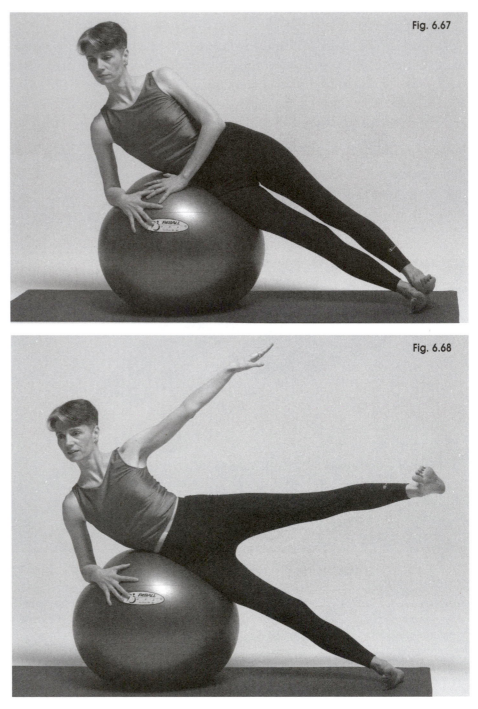

Fig. 6.67

Fig. 6.68

the shoulders. Use the arm that is on the ball to lift you taller. Press the side edge of your foot into the mat (fig. 6.67).
3. When you are ready, flex the top foot and lift the leg and the arm (fig. 6.68). Hold the position and breathe naturally.
4. Return the leg and arm and repeat three times. Change sides.

Ports de Bras

This graceful exercise should be done slowly and smoothly to avoid motion sickness. You will be sweeping your arm around as you stretch your body back and look at the four corners of the room. Your head (and your gaze) will move with the motion of the arm, but the hips remain squared to the front.

Purpose To create a flowing movement outward from a secure center.

Watchpoints • Work slowly and smoothly to avoid motion sickness. • Keep hips squared to the front.

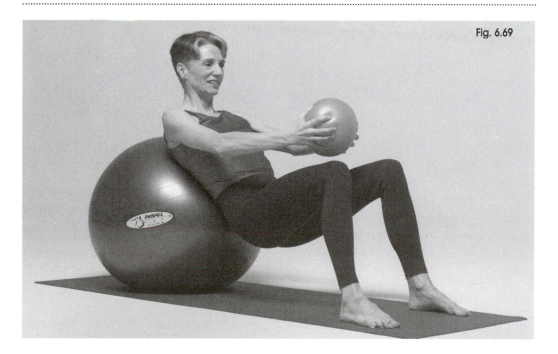

Fig. 6.69

starting position

Sit on your ball. Step your feet forward, bend at the hips and knees, and sink into a squat position. Your feet should be shoulder-distance apart. Hold the small ball at heart level (fig. 6.69).

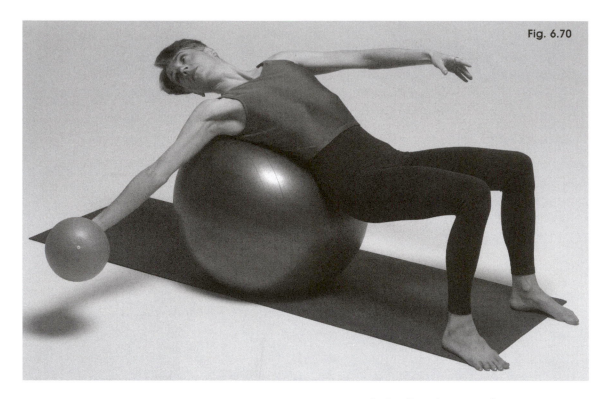

Fig. 6.70

movement: ports de bras

1. Inhale and sweep the arm back, following the small ball with your eyes. Stretch back so you look at one corner of the room (fig. 6.70).

2. Exhale and continue the motion, reaching the arm back until you are looking directly at the wall behind you (fig. 6.71).

3. Continue to sweep the arm so you look at the other corner. The body will rotate into a sidebend (fig. 6.72).

4. Return to the starting position. Inhale and reverse the direction of the circle.

5. Perform three circles to each side, slow and smooth.

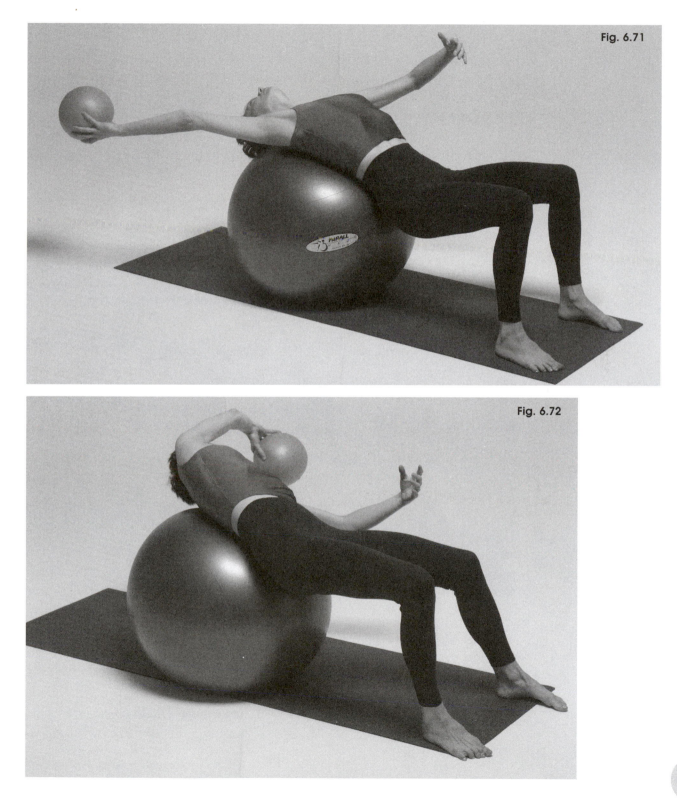

Fig. 6.71

Fig. 6.72

Plank with Hands on the Ball

In all exercises where we bear weight on the hands, it is very important that the shoulders remain down and relaxed and that the shoulder blades remain tight against the ribs and do not protrude or "wing" away from the rib cage. A plank or push-up with the hands resting on a ball is much more challenging than on a stable surface. Keep the body as stiff as a board and use a strong navel-to-spine connection to avoid sagging in the midriff. For more control place the ball against a wall.

Purpose To work the deep core and the upper body, and to strengthen balancing skills.

Watchpoints • Do not let the hips sag. • The elbows should angle back at a diagonal. • In movement 2 do not hyperextend your arms as you straighten them.

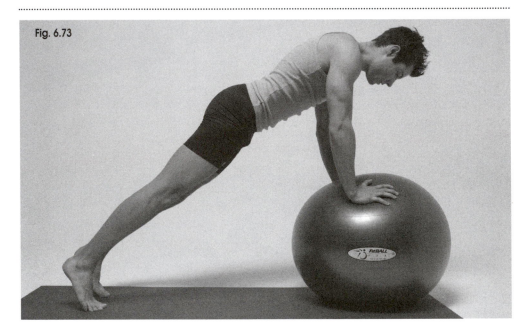

Fig. 6.73

starting position

Kneel in front of the ball. Place your hands on the ball shoulder-width apart. Step one leg back and then the other until you are in a very strong plank position. The abdominals are engaged (fig. 6.73).

movement 1: plank

1. Keep the body very still and hold for a number of seconds.
2. Rest and repeat three times, holding the pose longer each time.

movement 2: add push-up

1. Inhale to bend your elbows, lowering your chest to the ball.
2. Exhale to extend your elbows.
3. Inhale lower. Exhale extend.
4. Repeat eight times.

Kneel on the Ball

Practice makes perfect with this formidable balance exercise. All the muscles in the core must work or you cannot keep control. Start by straddling the ball, hugging the ball with your inner thighs and lifting your feet off the ground. Then graduate to balancing on your hands and knees. From there slowly lift up. When you are upright, gently squeeze the buttocks and keep the tailbone dropped. Make sure the space around you is completely clear of objects in case you lose balance. You may want to have someone spot you at first.

Purpose To challenge core and balance.

Watchpoint • Master one step before you move to the next. Do not grip the ball with your feet. Feet should ideally be off the ball. Work in a large empty space.

starting position

Stand behind the ball and place hands shoulder-distance apart on the top of the ball.

movement 1: hands and knees on the ball

1. Taking your time, slowly shift your weight onto the ball so that only your toes are dangling on the mat. Knees are slightly apart.
2. When you are ready, lift your toes from the mat and hold in the kneeling position for a number of seconds (fig. 6.74). Hold steady for as long as possible.
3. Repeat three to five times.

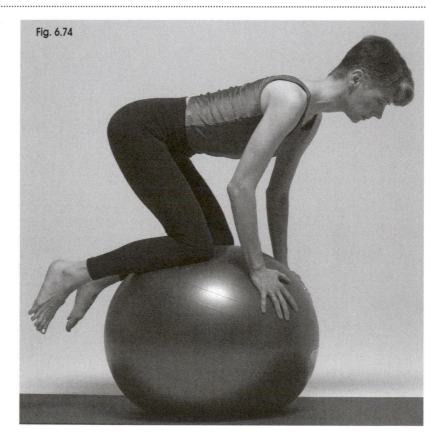

Fig. 6.74

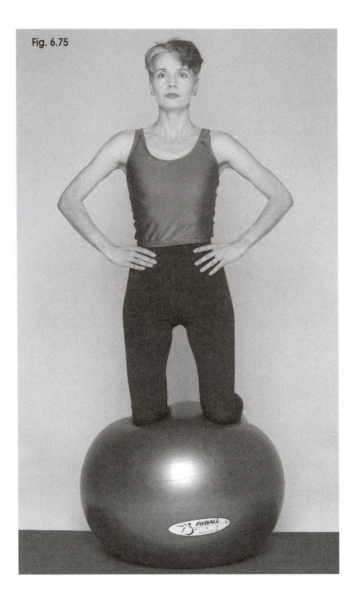

Fig. 6.75

movement 2: kneel on the ball

1. After practicing movement 1 for a while, begin by slowly lifting the upper body.

2. Stretch up tall, hands on your hips. Keep the tailbone dropped (fig. 6.75). Breathe naturally and hold for as long as possible.

3. To come down, place the hands on the ball, roll the ball backward, and place the feet on the mat.

4. Repeat three to five times.

7

The Short Workouts

The short workouts that follow are complete sessions in themselves, but for balanced fitness they need to be complemented by a stretching program, aerobic conditioning, and strength training.

When selecting a short Abs on the Ball workout choose the level you are realistically at. Begin your abs training by attempting one fifteen-minute workout per day, or one thirty-minute workout three or four times a week. Keep to the order presented here, building up pace and intensity without sacrificing form. Eventually you should move smoothly from one exercise to the next without stopping; this approach builds endurance and the sense of flow important to all Pilates-based work. Even if you are doing the same short workout every day, try to find something fresh in each movement. Abs on the Ball is very textured work—concentration and focus will help you discover new layers.

If you are training for a particular sport, the fifteen-minute basic-level abs workout can be used as a warm-up. The intermediate and advanced short workouts, however, can fatigue the core. Save them for training days.

Each short workout here has been delineated by time and level. The page numbers allow you to cross-reference back to the full instructions; the photos provide quick visual reference. Perform six to eight repetitions of each move unless otherwise indicated.

Schedule workouts into your routine to keep you on track. Sooner than you think you will notice significant changes in your posture, the fit of your clothes, and, most important of all, how you feel in your body. Enjoy Abs on the Ball and tell others about the secret to your success!

Fifteen-minute Basic Abs Workout

Practicing the Fundamentals (pp. 19–29)

1. back breathing

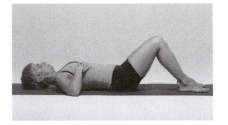

2. neutral pelvis lying on the mat

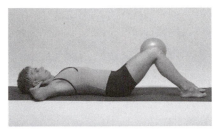

3. lifting the head off the mat

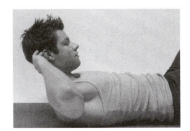

(gaze is on your knees, not on the ceiling)

4. finding the pelvic floor

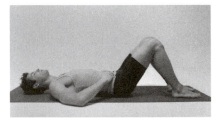

(imagine the pelvic floor gently drawing upward and tightening)

5. feel the transversus abdominis

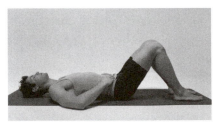

(place your fingers one inch in from hip bones to feel the pressure as the pelvic floor contracts)

Ab Curls with Small Ball (p. 30)

6. ab curls

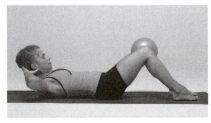

(use exhalation to gently sink navel and lift the head)

Half Roll-up with Arm Stretch and Tabletop Legs (p. 32)

7. without arm stretch

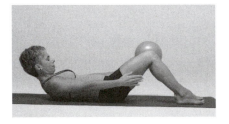

8. with arm stretch

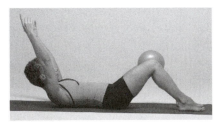

(keep one hand behind head if you have neck strain)

Small Extensions on Small Ball (p. 35)

9. connecting navel to spine

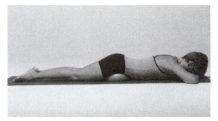

(use a very soggy ball under the pelvis)

10. single leg extensions

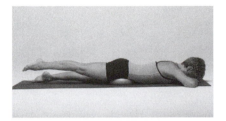

11. shell stretch

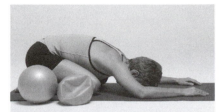

(with knee problems do Side Shell)

Half Roll Down (p. 38)

12. half roll down

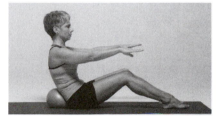

(maintain C-curve by keeping navel pulled in)

13. half roll down with obliques

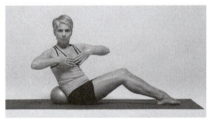

Rolling like a Ball (p. 40)

14. without rolling back

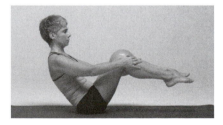

15. rolling like a ball

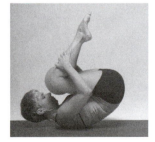

Single Leg Stretch (p. 42)

16. head down or lifting the head

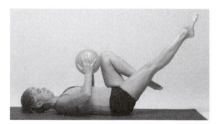

(keep legs high if you have low-back pain)

Oblique Twists (p. 45)

17. oblique twist

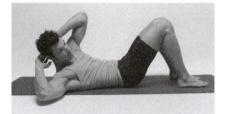

(keep pelvis stable and anchored in neutral position)

18. just squeeze

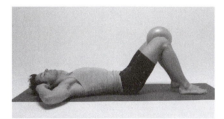

(don't let the tail curl up when you squeeze)

Ab Curls on Small Ball (p. 51)

19. ab curls

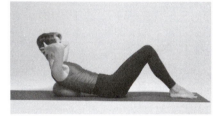

(sink the navel and keep pelvis in neutral)

20. add oblique twist

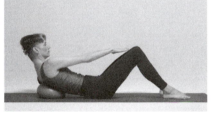

(eight times on the same side, then repeat on the other side)

Hip Rolls with Small Ball (p. 49)

21. ordinary hip roll

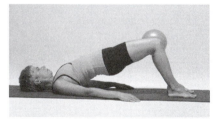

(imagine vertebrae moving individually)

22. with arm stretch

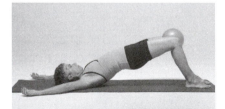

(buttocks squeeze together; pelvic floor is engaged)

Thirty-minute Basic Abs Workout

Practicing the Fundamentals (pp. 19–29)

1. side breathing

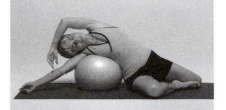

(both sides)

2. neutral pelvis lying on the mat

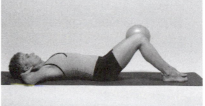

3. connecting navel to spine

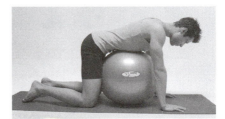

(hold contraction for 10 seconds, breathing naturally)

4. add hand lifts and contraction

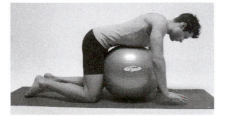

5. pelvic floor elevator exercise

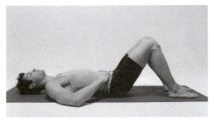

(pause on each of three "floors" for a contraction of 5 to 10 seconds)

Ab Curls with Small Ball (p. 30)

6. ab curls

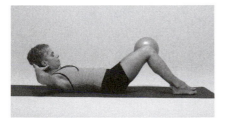

Half Roll-up with Arm Stretch and Tabletop Legs (p. 32)

7. with arm stretch

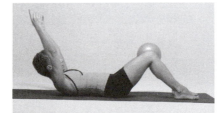

8. add tabletop legs

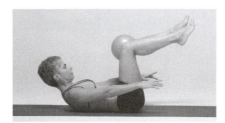

(keep legs close to body until you become stronger)

Small Extensions on Small Ball (p. 35)

9. connecting navel to spine

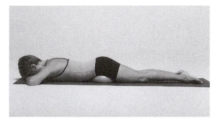

10. small extension

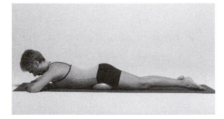

11. single leg extension

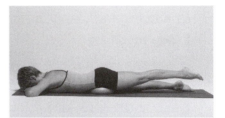

12. single arm extension

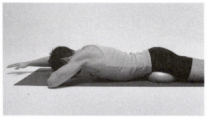

13. shell stretch

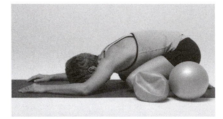

(repeat on same side five times and
then change arms)

Half Roll Down (p. 38)

14. half roll down

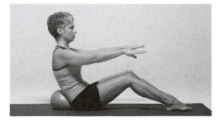

(watch for bulging abdominals—
a sure sign the deep connection is lost)

15. half roll down with obliques

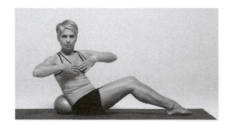

Rolling like a Ball (p. 40)

16. rolling like a ball

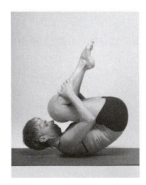

Single Leg Stretch *(p. 42)*

17. passing the ball under the leg   **18. with small ball support**

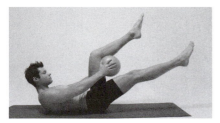 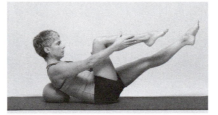

Oblique Twists *(p. 45)*

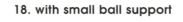

19. oblique twist   **20. just squeeze**   **21. check in with the deep abdominals**

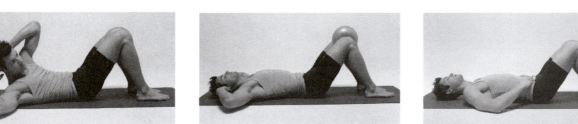

Sidework with Small Ball *(p. 47)*

22. thigh squeeze   **23. press top leg**

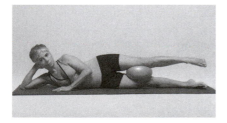 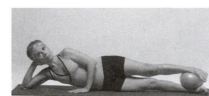

24. ankle squeeze and lift   **25. inner thigh circles**

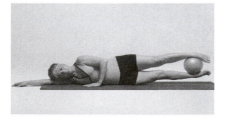 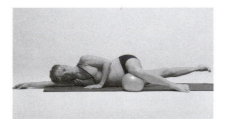

(repeat Sidework on both sides)

The Waterfall (p. 53)

26. the waterfall

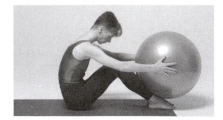

(avoid with low-back pain)

Hips Rolls on Large Ball (p. 55)

27. ordinary hip roll

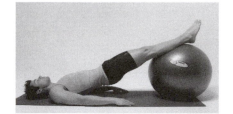

28. hold pelvis in air

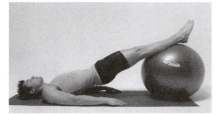

(hold pelvis steady for 15 to 20 seconds, breathing naturally)

Hip Rolls with Balance (p. 56)

29. lift wrists

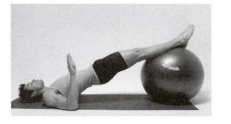

30. lift head

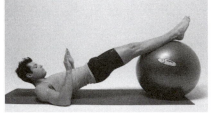
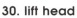

(do not overarch at the top by lifting the pelvis too high; breathe naturally)

Ball Balance (p. 65)

31. using the wall

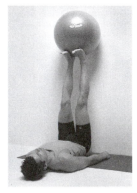

(use a small ball under the hips for tightness in low back or hamstrings)

Walk Up and Down (p. 61)

32. fingers on the ball

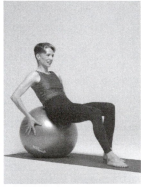

(use a sticky mat or rubber-soled shoes; when ready add speed)

33. hands off the ball

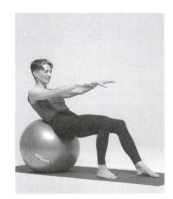

Rolling from Side to Side (p. 64)

34. roll from side to side

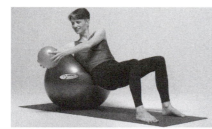

(keep pelvis square to the front)

Ab Curls on Large Ball (p. 58)

35. hips up

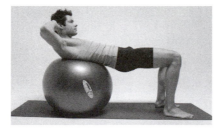

(eight repetitions on one side, then switch sides)

36. oblique variation

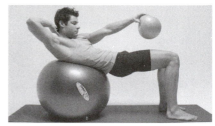

Hip Rolls with Leg Extension (p. 50)

37. stretch out back and abdominals

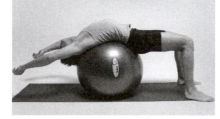

(avoid with low-back pain)

38. ordinary hip roll

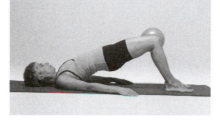

39. with leg extension

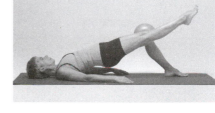

Body Openers (p.114)

40. upper chest opener

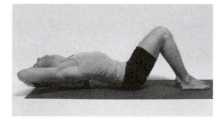

41. upper chest opener with twist

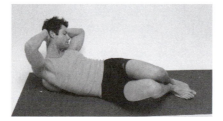

Fifteen-minute Intermediate Abs Workout

Practicing the Fundamentals (pp. 19–29, 68–74)

1. finding the core sitting

2. lift toes / lift leg and extend

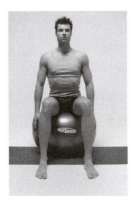
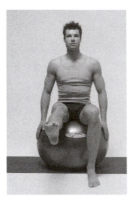

(hold deep connection for 10 to 25 seconds, rest for 10 to 25 seconds.)

3. back breathing

4. pelvic floor elevator exercise

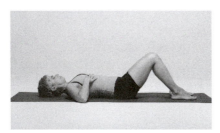
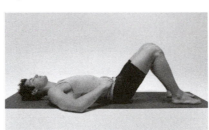

Ab Curls with Small Ball (p. 30)

5. ab curls

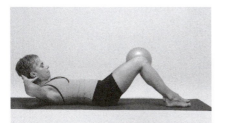

The Waterfall (p. 53)

6. the waterfall

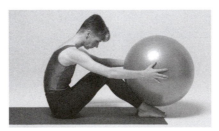

(avoid with low-back pain)

Full Roll-up (p. 75)

7. the full roll-up

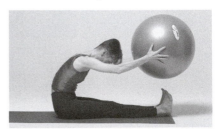

(avoid with low-back pain)

Rolling like a Ball (p. 40)

8. with large ball

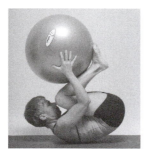

Double Leg Stretch (p. 77)

9. with small ball support

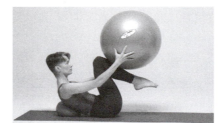

10. without small ball support

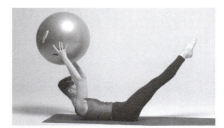

(keep head on mat if you have neck tension)

Lower and Lift (p. 82)

11. lower and lift

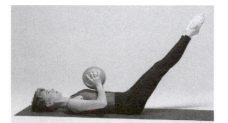

(keep low back on mat; do not use momentum)

Spine Twist (p. 86)

12. bend knees

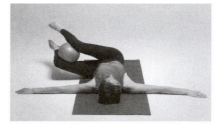

Leg Circles, Bicycle, and Scissors in Air (p. 88)

13. open and close

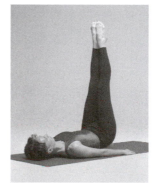

(use navel-to-spine connection to keep low back anchored on the ball)

14. leg circles

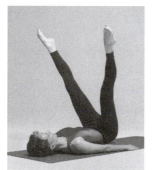

(both directions)

15. scissors in air

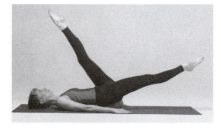

16. bicycle in air

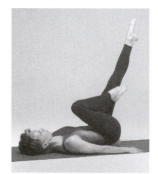

(five "pedal strokes" in one direction, then reverse the direction)

Thigh and Ankle Squeeze and Supported Swan (p. 93)

17. thigh squeeze

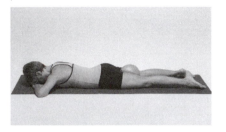

18. squeeze ball at ankles

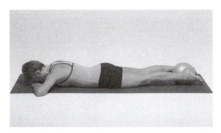

19. lift ball and squeeze

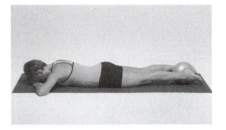

20. the cat

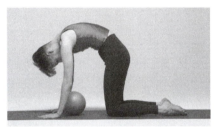

On Elbows (p. 91)

21. bend and stretch legs

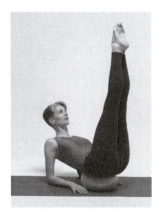

22. open and close legs

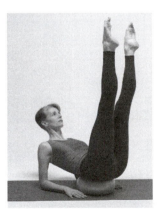

(don't sink between the shoulders)

Back Extensions on Knees (p. 101)

23. on knees

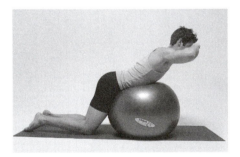

Side Shell with Kick (p. 106)

24. without kick

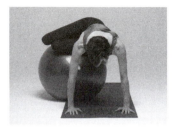

25. with kick

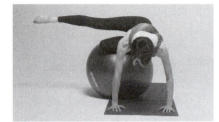

(make sure ball is in proper position
before you roll up into Shell)

26. shell on the ball

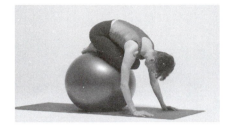

Thirty-minute Intermediate Abs Workout

Practicing the Fundamentals (pp. 19–29, 68–74)

1. single knee lift stabilizing exercise

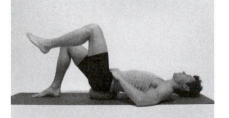

(slowly lift and lower leg, keeping the
abdominal connection)

2. double knee lift stabilizing exercise

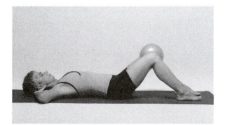

3. side breathing

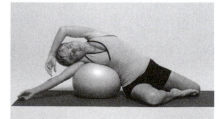

(both sides)

4. neutral pelvis lying on the mat

Ab Curls with Small Ball (p. 30)

5. ab curls

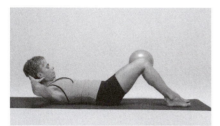

6. hold contraction

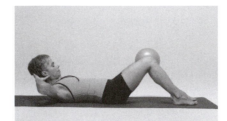

(hold for three seconds)

The Waterfall (p. 53)

7. the waterfall

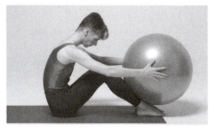

(avoid with low-back pain)

Full Roll-up (p. 75)

8. the full roll-up

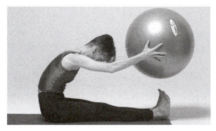

(avoid with low-back pain)

Double Leg Stretch (p. 77)

9. without small ball support

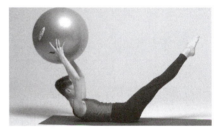

Teaser Prep (p. 79)

10. feet on the mat

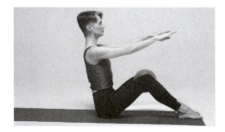

11. legs in the air

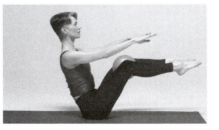

Leg Pull-up and Bicycle (p. 84)

12. leg pull-up

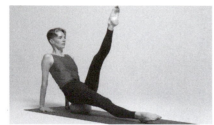

(three kicks each side)

13. sitting-on-the-ball bicycle

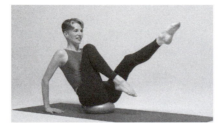

(work for a few counts in one direction, then reverse direction)

14. V-shaped legs

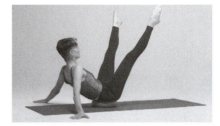

(place hands wider on the mat and shift weight slightly back)

Spine Twist (p. 86)

15. bend knees

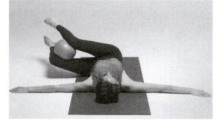

(squeeze abdominals as you bring the heavy legs through center)

16. straight legs

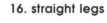
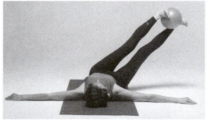

Thigh and Ankle Squeeze and Supported Swan (p. 93)

17. thigh squeeze

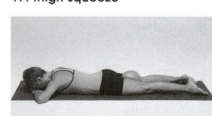

18. lift ball and squeeze

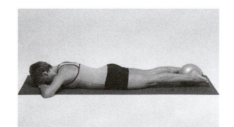

19. bend knees and squeeze

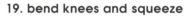
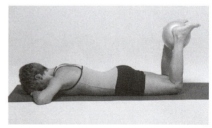

20. supported swan

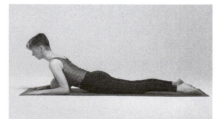

21. the cat

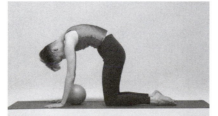

(don't sink between the shoulders)

175

Bend and Stretch (p. 96)

22. bend and stretch

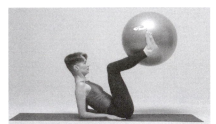

23. with ball twist

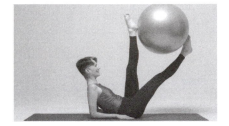

(keep legs 45 degrees or higher
in both exercises)

Backward Crunch (p. 98)

24. backward crunch

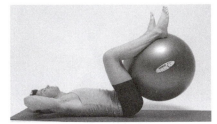

(keep low back pressed down as you
raise hips slightly off mat)

Hip Rolls with Balance (p. 56)

25. hold pelvis in air

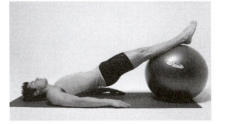

26. lift wrists

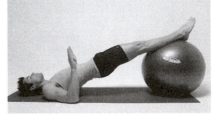

27. lift head

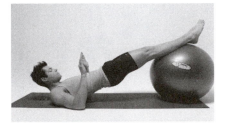

Hip Lift (p.99)

28. hip lift

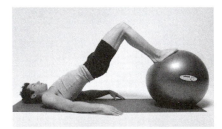

(repeat three times and try on small ball)

29. stretch hamstrings

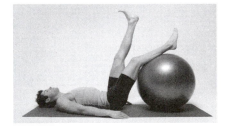

Ball Balance (p. 65)

30. away from the wall

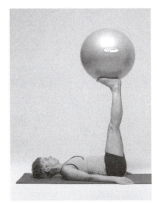

176

Side Raises (p. 102)

31. side raises

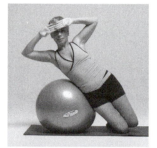

(keep body "stiff as a board";
work both sides)

Side Crunches (p. 103)

32. hands across chest

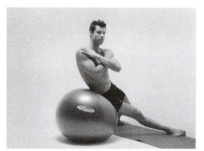

(use wall to stabilize your feet;
work both sides)

Planks
(p. 104)

33. both feet on the ball

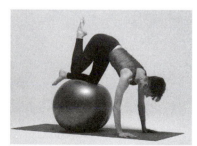

**34. lift one foot or lift
foot to side**

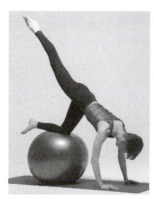

(engage deep abdominals to protect low back and keep body from sagging)

Back Extensions on
Knees (p.101)

35. on knees

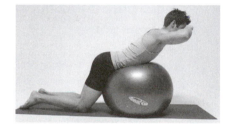

(repeat both sides)

Arabesque (p. 108)

36. the stork

(repeat two to three times on both
sides)

37. the arabesque

(repeat two to three times on
both sides)

Tabletop Balance (p. 112)

38. tabletop balance

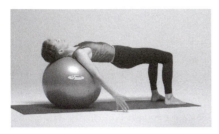

39. take hands off

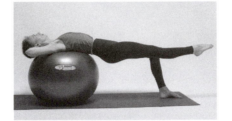

40. stretch out back and abdominals

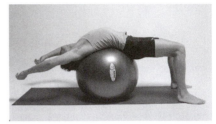

Fifteen-minute Advanced Abs Workout

Practicing the Fundamentals (pp. 19–29, 68–74, 117–121)

1. one leg standing: the kite

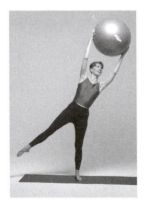

2. one leg standing: the tree

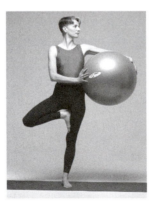

3. feet on one or two small balls

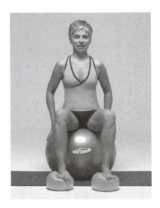

4. knee lift stabilizing exercise on small ball

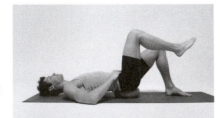

Ab Curls with Small Ball (p. 30)

5. ab curls

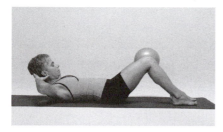

The Hundred (p. 122)

6. the hundred

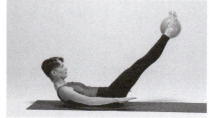

(squeeze gently on exhalation)

Full Roll-up (p. 75)

7. the full roll-up

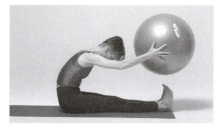

Rolling Like a Ball (p. 40)

8. with large ball

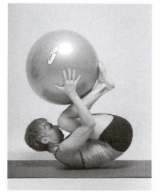

Double Leg Stretch (p. 77)

9. without small ball support

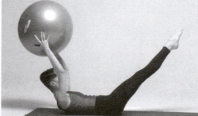

Roll Over (p. 123)

10. large or small ball at ankles

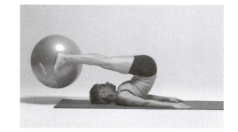

(do not take your weight so far back that you are crushing the neck; avoid with neck or low-back problems)

Side Bridge on Small Ball (p. 130)

11. side bridge

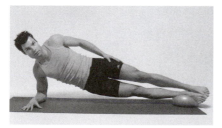

(hold for 5 to 10 seconds; repeat on other side)

Rocking Horse Extension (p. 135)

12. connecting navel to spine

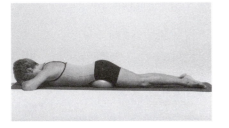

13. small extension

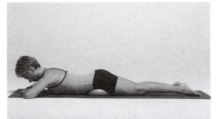

14. rocking horse extension

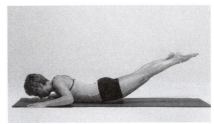

15. shell stretch

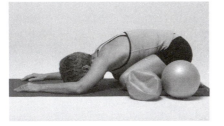

Scissors (p. 137)

16. scissors

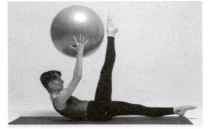

Teaser (p. 139)

17. straight legs in air

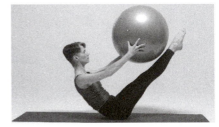

(can be done with small or large ball)

Sidebend and Twist (p. 142)

18. sidebend

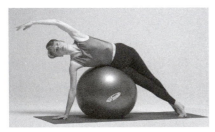

(avoid both movements with wrist, shoulder, or neck problems)

19. add twist

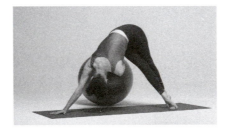

(repeat twice and change sides)

The Pike (p. 148)

20. the pike

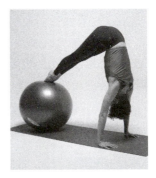

Tabletop Balance (p.112)

21. tabletop balance

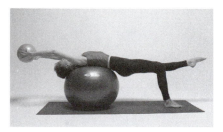

Planks (p. 104)

22. lift one foot or lift foot to side

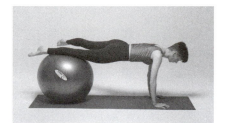

23. shell on the ball

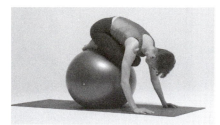

Thirty-minute Advanced Abs Workout

Practicing the Fundamentals (pp. 19–29, 68–74, 117–121)

1. neutral spine sitting

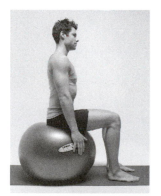

2. finding the core sitting

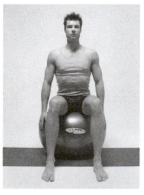

3. lift toes / lift leg and extend

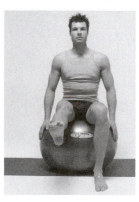

4. opposite hand and foot, two inches

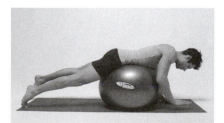

5. opposite hand and foot, full height

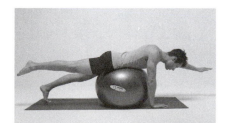

6. back breathing

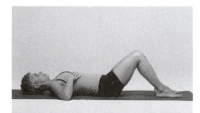

The Hundred (p. 122)

7. the hundred

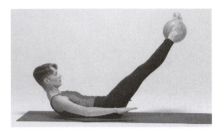

Single Leg Stretch (p. 42)

8. lifting the head

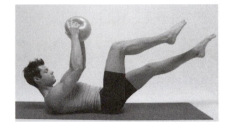

9. passing the ball under the leg

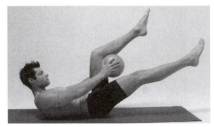

Spine Twist (p. 86)

10. bend knees

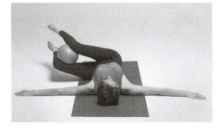

11. straight legs

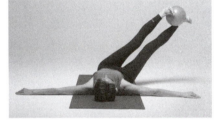

Corkscrew (p. 126)

12. with small ball support

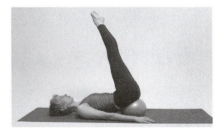

(keep circles small to begin with)

13. full corkscrew

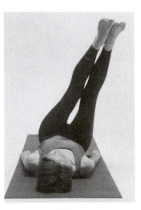

(three repetitions in each direction, alternating the direction of the circle; do corkscrew prep if you're not ready for full corkscrew)

Rocking Horse Extension (p. 135)

14. small extension

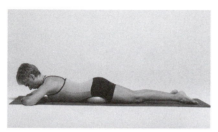

15. rocking horse extension

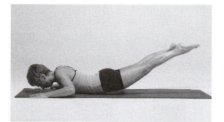

16. shell stretch

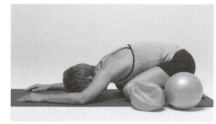

Boomerang (p. 132)

17. the boomerang

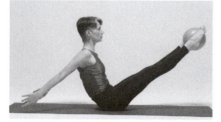

(keep knees bent if necessary)

On Elbows (p. 91)

18. bend and stretch legs

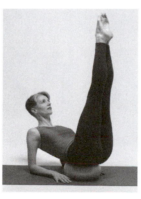

19. open and close legs

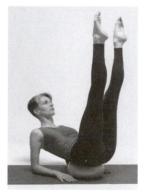

Leg Pull-up and Bicycle (p. 84)

20. leg pull-up or sitting-on-the-ball bicycle

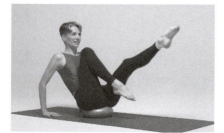

21. V-shaped legs

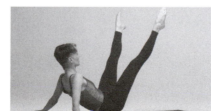

The Waterfall (p. 53)

22. the waterfall

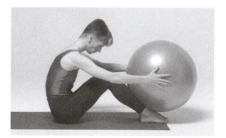

Full Roll-up (p. 75)
23. the full roll-up

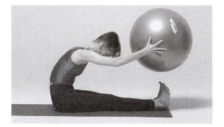

Double Leg Stretch (p. 77)
24. double leg stretch

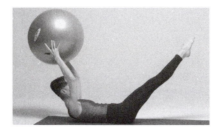

Scissors (p. 137)
25. scissors

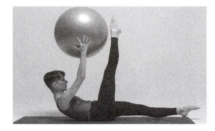

Teaser (p. 139)
26. straight legs in air or legs on the mat

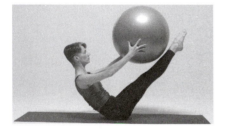

Bend and Stretch (p. 96)
27. with ball twist

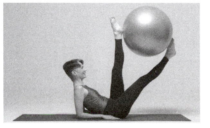

Hip Lift (p. 99)
28. hip lift on large or small ball

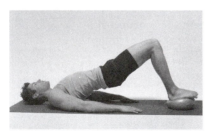

29. stretch hamstrings

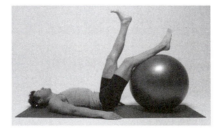

Side-twist Plank (p. 146)

30. side-twist plank

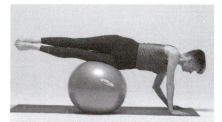

(keep legs straight and body
"stiff as a board")

Single Leg Shell (p. 149)

31. single leg shell

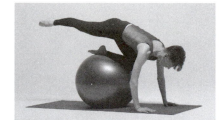

32. shell on the ball

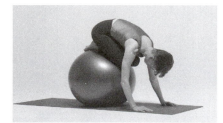

Kneeling Side Lifts (p. 151)

33. lower and lift

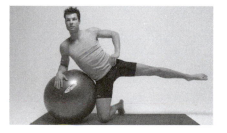

34. little circles

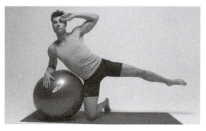

(Imagine you are circling from the hip
sockets, not the ankle)

Ab Curls on Large Ball (p. 58)

35. hips up

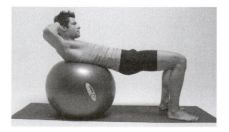

36. oblique variation

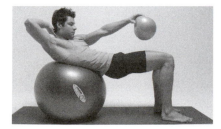

Ports de Bras (p. 155)

37. ports de bras

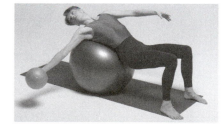

(keep this movement slow and
smooth to prevent motion sickness)

The Star (p. 153)

38. the star

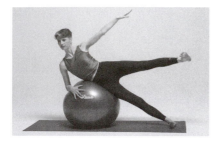

Plank with Hands on the Ball (p. 158)

39. plank, or add push-up

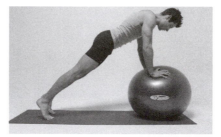

Kneel on the Ball (p. 159)

40. hands and knees on the ball

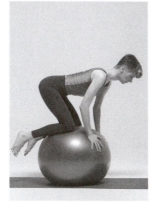

(master one level before moving to the next)

41. kneel on the ball

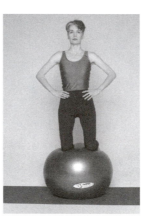

42. stretch out back and abdominals

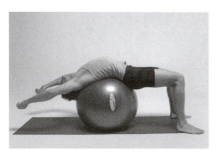

Resources

Books

Craig, Colleen. *Pilates on the Ball*. Rochester, Vt: Healing Arts Press, 2001.

Creager, Caroline. *Bounce Back into Shape After Baby*. Berthoud, Colo.: Executive Physical Therapy, Inc., 2001.

Goldenberg, Lorne, and Peter Twist. *Strength Ball Training*. Champaign, Ill.: Human Kinetics, 2002.

Jemmett, Richard. *Spinal Stabilization: The New Science of Back Pain*. Halifax: RMJ Fitness and Rehabilitation Consultants, 2002.

Linford, Monica. Awaken Your Body, Balance Your Mind: Chi Ball Method. London: Thorsons, 2000.

McGill, Stuart. *Low Back Disorders: Evidence-based Prevention and Rehabilitation*. Champaign, Ill: Human Kinetics, 2002.

Posner-Mayer, Joanne. *Swiss Ball Applications for Orthopedic and Sports Medicine*. Longmont, Colo.: Ball Dynamics International, Inc., 1995.

Richardson, Carolyn, Gwendolen Jull, Julie Hides, and Paul Hodges. *Therapeutic Exercise for Spinal Segmental Stabilization in Low Back Pain*. London: Churchill Livingstone, 1999.

Robinson, Lynne, and Gordon Thomson. *Body Control the Pilates Way*. London: Boxtree, 1997.

Searle, Sally, and Cathy Meeus. *Secrets of Pilates*. New York: DK Publishing Inc., 2001.

Ungaro, Alycea. *Pilates Body in Motion*. New York: DK Publishing Inc., 2002.

Siler, Brooke. *The Pilates Body*. New York: Broadway Books, 2000.

Stott-Merrithew, Moira, and Beth Evans. *Comprehensive Matwork Manual*. Toronto: Merrithew Corporation, 2001.

Winsor, Mari. *The Pilates Powerhouse*. Cambridge, Mass.: Perseus Books, 1999.

Zake, Yamuna, and Stephanie Golden. *Body Rolling: An Approach to Complete Muscle Release*. Rochester, Vt.: Healing Arts Press, 1997.

Exercise Ball Videotapes

Colleen Craig's On the Ball: An Innovative Ball Video Based on the Work of Joseph Pilates,
  VHS/Color/45 mins. www.pilatesontheball.com

Pilates Mini-Ball Workout with Leslee Bender, VHS/Color.

Paul Chek's Swiss Ball Exercises for Better Abs, Buns and Backs, VHS/Color/61 mins.

Exercises for the Pelvic Floor by Beate Carrière, VHS/Color/25 mins.

Fitball—Back to Functional Movement by Trish Scott, VHS/Color/30 mins.

Fitball—Upper Body Challenge and *Fitball—Lower Body Challenge*, by Cheryl Soleway,
  VHS/Color/45 mins. each.

Swiss Ball Applications for Orthopedic and Sports Medicine by Joanne Posner-Mayer,
  VHS/Color/90 mins.

The above videotapes can be ordered through Ball Dynamics International; see the following page for contact information. *Colleen Craig's On the Ball* video can be ordered through Know Your Body Best in Canada and Ball Dynamics International in the United States.

Ball and Video
Ordering Information

Ball Dynamics International, Inc.
Makers of Fitball®. Catalog of
exercise balls, videotapes, and
accessories. 800-752-2255.
www.fitball.com

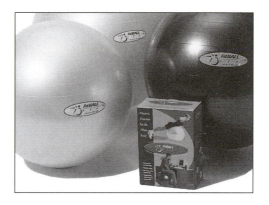

Know Your Body Best
Canadian distributor of
exercise balls, *Colleen Craig's
On the Ball* videotape,
therapeutic massage equipment
and supplies.
800-881-1681 (in Canada).
www.knowyourbodybest.com

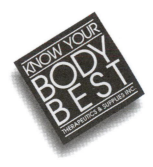

Acknowledgments

I have had the pleasure and great luck to work with outstanding teachers in my ongoing Pilates training. I would like to sincerely thank Moira Stott-Merrithew for exposing me to and certifying me in Stott Pilates. When I left Moira's extensive certification program and found myself teaching on my own I began to fully appreciate the intelligence of her contemporary approach. I have also learned much from other wonderful teachers and colleagues: Beth Evans, Mariane Braaf, Syl Klotz, Elaine Biagi-Turner, Connie Di Salvo, Mari Naumovski, and Danielle Belec. In addition there are those whose workshops, videos, books, or discussions I have found invaluable: Tanya Crowell, Frank Bach, Karen Carlson, Diane Woodruff, Cheryl Soleway, Paul Chek, Trish Scott, Caroline C. Creager, Leslee Bender, Miyuki Yamaguchi, Janet Davis, Janet Lemon, Esther Myers, Anne-Marie Hood, Laura Misek, Amah Heubi, Petra Dobesova, Katja Hambrecht, Irene Gerstner-Mühleck, Enrico Ceron, and Paola del Fabbro. The concepts behind Abs on the Ball were influenced by the teachings of Joseph Pilates and the research and wisdom of Rick Jemmett, Joanne Posner-Mayer, Stuart McGill, Carolyn Richardson, Gwendolen Jull, Paul Hodges, Julie Hides, and Beate Carrière.

I am very grateful to my sponsors and distributors who supplied the balls and for generously funding the photographs that appear in the book; in Canada, Donna Micallef and Constance Rennett and their hard-working staff at Know Your Body Best; in the States, Dayna Gutru and her associates at Ball Dynamics International. Many thanks to Daniella Smoller of Thera Med in South Africa, Trish Scott of IncrediBall Enterprises in Vancouver, and Nevio Cosani and Ledraplastic factory in Italy for inviting me to present my work.

I am grateful to Susan Lee of Canadian Personal Trainers Network and Mari Naumovski of BodySpheres who read and commented on earlier drafts of the manuscript. Many thanks to Claire Letemendia whose expert editorial assistance greatly helped shape and refine the manuscript. I am grateful to Marie Jover-Stapinski and Simon Fortin for appearing in the book with me. Thanks to David Hou for his wonderful photos and instructive illustrations and to Liz Robertson for makeup. Thanks to Paul Robinson at the University of Toronto Varsity Shop for generously supplying the clothing for both books and the video.

I would like to take this opportunity to thank Susan Davidson, my editor, and her collegues at Healing Arts Press, who so successfully launched *Pilates on the Ball* into the world. Susan especially made the publishing process for both books extremely gratifying. Her calm approach and expert guidance transformed two messy manuscripts into real and beautiful books. Thanks to Peri Champine for creating the sensational covers, Jon Graham for believing (with Susan) in *Pilates on the Ball*, Jeanie Levitan, Rob Meadows, and the rest of the design, production, and marketing teams at Healing Arts Press. I would also like to extend my thanks to Tara Persaud and Alan Zweig at Ten Speed Press; my agent, David Johnston; my accountant, John Chaplin; and Tony Yue at Creative Post. A special thanks to Marie Lussier for generously supplying me with legal services.

I am most grateful for the steady, loving support of my family and friends. Dominque Cardona and Laurie Colbert for volunteering to film my video; Lynne Viola (and Monty) for steadfast emotional support over the years; my parents, Lorraine and David Craig; sister, Jane Welch; and nieces, Lyndsey and Lauren. Finally, I am blessed with very loyal students and send them many, many thanks.

Books of Related Interest

Pilates on the Ball
The World's Most Popular Workout Using the Exercise Ball
by Colleen Craig

Yoga on the Ball
Enhance Your Yoga Practice Using the Exercise Ball
by Carol Mitchell

Body Rolling
An Experiential Approach to Complete Muscle Release
by Yamuna Zake and Stephanie Golden

The Five Tibetans
Five Dynamic Exercises for Health, Energy, and Personal Power
by Christopher S. Kilham

The Heart of Yoga
Developing a Personal Practice
by T. K. V. Desikachar

Rolfing
Reestablishing the Natural Alignment and Structural Integration
of the Human Body for Vitality and Well-Being
by Ida P. Rolf, Ph.D.

The Alexander Technique
How to Use Your Body without Stress
by Wilfred Barlow, M.D.

Offering from the Conscious Body
The Discipline of Authentic Movement
by Janet Adler

Inner Traditions • Bear & Company
P.O. Box 388 • Rochester, VT 05767 • 1-800-246-8648
www.InnerTraditions.com

Or contact your local bookseller